WILDERNESS MEDICINE

by

WILLIAM W. FORGEY, M.D.

Chairman, Emergency Medicine Department
Ross Clinic, Merrillville, Indiana
Teaching Affiliate in Clinical Pharmacy
Butler University, Indianapolis, Indiana
Member, Explorer's Club
New York City, New York

INDIANA CAMP SUPPLY BOOKS

Pittsboro, Indiana

WILDERNESS MEDICINE

Copyright © 1979 by William W. Forgey, M.D.

Published by
Indiana Camp Supply, Inc.,
405 Osborne, Pittsboro, IN 46167

Library of Congress Cataloging in Publication Data

Forgey, William W   1942 -
    Wilderness medicine.

    Bibliography: p.
    Includes index.
    1. Backpacking -- Accidents and injuries.
    2. First aid in illness and injury. 3. Wilderness survival. I. Title [DNLM: 1. Expeditions.
    2. First Aid. 3. Hygiene. 4. Travel. WA292.3
    F721]
    RC88.9.H55F67   614.8'8   79-89027

International Standard Book Number:
    0-934802-02-5 paper
    0-934802-03-3 hardback
Library of Congress Catalog Card Number: 79-89027

For Fred and Naomi Cook

Foreword

by Calvin Rutstrum

What essentially can I say as one of long wilderness experience, and as only a medical corpsman in the First World War, about a professionally compiled guide such as this for maintaining health beyond the ken of professional clinical help?

The answer is easy, as they say about a certain credit card: "Don't leave home without it!"

Much laymen fear of traveling deep in the wilds is that in the event of serious illness or accident, one might become helpless or die through lack of medical treatment. Every outgoing paddle stroke does, of course, bring one farther away from clinical help.

It may be said that the chief risk early in the trip is what contagion or potential illness one brings into the wilderness. One generally is not waylaid in the wilds by disease, stealthily lurking behind ambushes, but reasonable care from exposure, drinking water, and endemic disease must be taken. Potential accidents are a risk. Here, naturally, the best prophylaxis is care in one's physical movements. The important thing is to know what as layman one can do in the event of an accident.

In my wilderness travels to avoid complex celestial calculations in the field, I precomputed positions for various places and times, so that only a simple altitude reading checked my position. On the same premise, it is sensible to read, before one embarks on a trip, how one can take care of a clinical problem in the wilds should it be encountered. In a metaphorical sense, precompute your safety before you leave by reading this manual.

This does not mean that one has to memorize a vast amount of clinical data. The important thing is to understand the INSTANT REFERENCE CLINICAL INDEX from previous reading of this guide so that a quicker reference can be made to it when the emergency occurs.

The layman at times has to extend himself in clinical scope farther than what he might ordinarily find the need to do. Here some wisdom and caution needs to be exercised. For example, I was called to help in a wilderness area when an individual had a treble fishhook caught in the region close to his eye. For me, as a layman, to attempt removing the hook would risk possible loss of the eye, damage to a vital nerve, or some other difficulty. I simply immobilized the hook with a tape support to keep it from doing further damage until we could get plane transportation to fly him out for surgery.

Sometimes as amateur doctors we get too professional. I came upon a case of hemorrhage in a downtown office building, where anxious people were trying to stop the blood flow with a necktie as tourniquet. When I said, "Just put a cork in the bottle" and with a clean handkerchief simply put direct pressure on the wound until the ambulance arrived, the spectators thought me ill-advised until they saw it work.

One thus oscillates between unprofessionally doing too much or too little. With radio communications one can sometimes obtain information to treat a clinical problem from a doctor after he has received all objective and subjective symptoms, but rarely does one have this opportunity. This is where this book serves a vital function.

At one time I set up a private expedition and went to great lengths to have a physican make up the medical kit and advise the members how to use it. Weeks later the kit was returned unopened, no one having received so much as a scratch. This, of course, is the fortunate situation, and we can hope the Wilderness Expedition Medical Kit similarly gets returned home unused.

Thus we might warn: avoid the need for field treatment by being careful, but be prepared beforehand with enough knowledge for clinical emergencies should they occur. At least have the foresight to bring along information on what to do.

This volume ought to be diligently read! It could be the required data for assurring a successful wilderness journey.

Calvin Rutstrum

Calvin Rutstrum
Marine-on-St. Croix, Minnesota
1979

Acknowledgements

For the summation of experience that is so essential for the production of a book of this nature, I am grateful to individuals from two areas of specialized knowledge -- medicine and the ways of the wilderness. I have been fortunate to have worked closely over the last ten years with experts in both of these fields who have extended many courtesies to me in addition to knowledge. I particularly must acknowledge the help of Dean Robert R. Sturgeon of the College of Arts and Sciences, Indiana University, Bloomington, Indiana, and to Deans Steven C. Beering, M.D., George T. Lukemeyer, M.D., and James F. Carter, M.D. of the Indiana University School of Medicine, Indianapolis, Indiana, and to Robert M. Seibel, M.D., Nashville, Indiana. Sigurd F. Olson and Calvin Rutstrum have frequently aided me with technical and personal assistance in the execution of expeditions and acquisition of wilderness knowledge.

The real impetus for writing this book came from the many expedition leaders and woodsmen heading into isolation from medical care who requested my assistance in preparing medical kits, instruction, and TRAINING for their trips.

The Journal of the American Medical Association and the American Heart Association have granted permission to reproduce the CPR illustrations on pages 41 and 43 in this book from the "Cardiopulmonary Resuscitation Standards" published in JAMA, February 18, 1974, Vol. 227, No. 7, which is acknowledged with appreciation.

Grateful acknowledgement is made to Banyan International Corporation which graciously authorized the reproduction of illustrations of the needle cricothyrotomy technique from their manual, *The Banyan Emergency Reference Guide*, 1978, which appear on Pages 46 and 47 of this publication.

Special thanks is due to Dover Publications, Inc., New York City, who very kindly provided the illustrations for the cover of *WILDERNESS MEDICINE*.

All other illustrations in this book were prepared by James Ross, an unusually talented 19-year-old, who returned in January 1979 from a 7-month sojourn in the Canadian subarctic. These illustrations were prepared for publication by Victoria Bradfield, whose help in the general layout of this book was indispensable.

A particular debt of gratitude is owed to Jean Reder, who controlled the over-all production of this work.

I was sustained in this project by the encouragement of Fred and Naomi Cook, close friends without whose help *WILDERNESS MEDICINE* would not have been possible. Nick Nickels of Lakefield, Ontario, constantly kept me to the task, while my family tolerated the last nine months of nocturnal typewriter noise without complaint. To these people, my sincere appreciation and gratitude are extended.

Bill Forgey
Gary, Indiana
27 April 1979

INTRODUCTION

Whether backpacking, camping, climbing or canoeing -- the mastery of technique includes planning and carrying the lightest loads possible. With regard to a medical kit, the lightest load will only be possible with multifunctional components. Intelligent choice of type and quantity of bandaging material will also aid in reducing bulk and volume to proper amounts. The existence of a medical kit of some sort is well established as one of the ten essentials for even short hikes away from home base (along with fire-making equipment, canteen, knife, flashlight, map and compass, extra protective clothing and sunglasses).

A very lightweight, multipurpose prescription medical kit has formed the basis for this book. Each of the components is multifunctional, thus saving weight, bulk and cost for the expedition.

Although pre-trip training and study are necessary, familiarization with the short list of primary medications is also made simple. This kit is so complete that it is adequate for use during prolonged periods of isolation where medical evacuation to outside help is virtually impossible. Many close-to-home outdoorsmen will also benefit from the complete discussions of wilderness related medical problems.

Many fine products that do not require prescriptions are available for medical treatment. A medical kit comprised of only these items is also described, with dosage amounts for normal OTC (Over-the-counter) usage and wilderness emergency usage explained.These components can be purchased over the counter in drugstores anywhere or through many outfitters such as the publisher.

All problems discussed in this book presuppose that the traveler has no professional medical help available and that he has access to either the prescription kit or nonprescription kit described. Full instructions are provided for therapy with each. Frequently, instructions are given for handling a particular problem with less than the above kits available -- the so-called "survival" situation with no medical kit. Conversely, where the drug of choice differs from the one available in the prescription kit, that drug and its use are also described. This has expanded the size of this book somewhat, but many disease states can be anticipated due to the geographical location about to be entered, and this listing of specific therapy may make medical planning much more logical for that particular expedition.

Although separate chapters describe both the prescription and nonprescription wilderness medical kit, a summary of both kits with brief treatment outline is reprinted in the centerfold on water resistant paper. This centerfold may be removed and packed with the medical kits to be used as a lightweight reference guide.

IMPORTANT!

IT SHOULD BE NOTED THAT TWO DIFFERENT MEDICAL KITS ARE DESCRIBED IN THIS BOOK. IF POSSIBLE, EQUIP YOURSELF WITH THE PRESCRIPTION MEDICAL KIT AND FOLLOW THE GUIDELINES FOR THERAPY INDICATED IN THIS BOOK AND THE SPECIFIC INSTRUCTIONS OF YOUR DOCTOR. IF NECESSARY, THE NONPRESCRIPTION (OTC or nonRx) MEDICAL KIT WILL PROVIDE REASONABLE THERAPY AS LONG AS THE GUIDELINES FOR USE LISTED BY THE MANUFACTURER ARE FOLLOWED AND THE INSTRUCTIONS INDICATED IN THIS BOOK ARE UNDERSTOOD AND CAREFULLY FOLLOWED AFTER CONSULTATION WITH YOUR DOCTOR.

EITHER ONE KIT OR THE OTHER NEED BE USED. WHILE INSTRUCTIONS FOR TREATMENT WITH BOTH KITS IS LISTED UNDER EACH SECTION, THERAPY SHOULD BE IMPLEMENTED WITH MEDICATIONS FROM ONE KIT OR THE OTHER — *NOT FROM BOTH AT THE SAME TIME.*

For example, I will frequently state something to the effect that "to treat the pain found with this condition, from the Rx kit use Tylenol #3, one tablet every 4 hours. From the nonRx kit use Percogesic, two tablets every 4 hours." This does not mean that both medications should be given. Give one OR the other, depending upon whether you are carrying the prescription (Rx) medical kit or the nonprescription (nonRx or OTC) medical kit.

PRE-TRIP MEDICAL TRAINING

Those contemplating medical/surgical responsibility for major expeditions, where one would not anticipate the capability of medical evacuation or availability of professional medical assistance, should familiarize themselves with every piece of equipment and the techniques required for their proper use prior to departure. As a rule, one should be able to find an outing club with a physician who is sympathetic to your requirements. Your family physician may not be a wilderness traveller, but he may be willing to advise on the techniques mentioned in this book. First aid courses are usually available in every community. If in doubt, contact your local Boy Scout Council, which should have knowledge of a physician with an outdoor lean.

Basic skills should certainly include a course in Cardio-pulmonary Resuscitation (CPR) and the general method of treating shock. In addition, it would behoove the group medic to have adequate knowledge of the following:

Signs, prevention and treatment of "thermal injury," to wit:
    Hypothermia
    Frostbite
    Burns
    Hyperthermia
Prevention and treatment of blisters (friction), abrasions and cuts
Prevention and treatment of animal bites, snake bites, scorpion bites and other zoogenic trauma peculiar to the area of anticipated operation.
Prevention and treatment of poison plant dermatitis
Properly acquiring and treating potable water; human waste disposal
Recognizing and treating High Altitude Illness
Immobilization splinting
When and how to evacuate
Medical treatment of anaphylaxis (shock from bee stings, etc.)

Although these subjects are discussed in this book, it should be stressed that CPR is certainly a skill that must be learned and practiced under supervision in order to be properly implemented during a time of need. It will be impractical to practice some of the skills discussed in this book, but there is no excuse for *everyone* not becoming CPR qualified.

PRE-TRIP PREPARATION/ PHYSICALS

Besides obtaining expedition members, equipment, food and designing a realistic route and time schedule, physical conditioning and pre-trip dental and medical physical examinations for all trip members make common sense. The dental exam should be made well in advance of the trip, thus allowing adequate time for possible needed corrections. The pre-trip physical should include attention to immunization schedules that vary, depending upon the region of the world to be visited (See Appendix), but as a minimum, each trip member should have a tetanus booster within the previous five to ten years.

Base line resting pulse rate, blood pressure and urinalysis should be determined for each member. Examination for a hernia or any tendency to form a hernia ought to be noted (such as a loose inguinal ring in males.)

An eye examination should have been performed within the previous three years upon everyone. For those over forty years of age I recommend an exam (including glaucoma check) within the previous year.

A prostate exam upon all men over forty and a Pap smear upon all females taking birth control pills or those over the age of forty should have been performed within the previous year. Cardiac stress testing (treadmill) is not required in persons with no symptoms of angina.

MEDICAL KITS

For a day hike away from camp (or car) a very light kit would reasonably consist of 6 Percogesic tablets (they come sealed in plastic), 5 butterfly bandages, 3 bandades (1" x 3" plastic strips) and a 1½ gram foil packet of triple antibiotic ointment (neomycin-bacitracin-polymyxin B). These items are readily available through several outfitters or through a pharmacy without prescription. They would care for cuts, burns, abrasions, blisters, fever, pain, muscle spasm, insomnia, even anxiety and itching. (Percogesic works wonders on stopping an itch, which is a type of pain stimulus). Yet, they are light enough not to encumber the carrier with bulk or weight. These items can be slipped into a canteen cover and kept there, so as not to be forgotten when that particular essential is picked up while departing.

The prescription wilderness medical kit which follows is adequate for up to ten persons in isolation for one to three months. Obviously, for a week long hike the quantities of bandaging material and medication can be scaled down.

The key element in any medical kit design is "multifunctional components." This has been achieved to a high degree with the prescription kit. For example, Phenergan tablets act to control nausea, allergic reactions, act as both sleeping pills and an antianxiety agent and increase the effectiveness of pain medication, depending upon the dosage. The antibiotic chosen has very wide latitude of use. The pain medication would alleviate fever, diarrhea, abdominal cramping, coughing and help eliminate itching. And so forth.

THE PRESCRIPTION (Rx) WILDERNESS EXPEDITION MEDICAL KIT

This kit should be adequate for two to ten persons on a trip into isolated areas lasting from one to three months. the BASIC KIT contains the essential items, while the AUGMENTATION KIT adds depth to the basic kit, notably the ability to suture lacerations and otherwise take care of trauma with more sophistication.

The basic portion of the Prescription Wilderness Expedition Medical Kit can be used to treat nearly every emergency condition listed in this book. The total weight of the basic portion of the kit is 13½ ounces. The augmentation portion weighs an additional 16 ounces. The total kit would thus weigh 29½ ounces using the largest number of the above items indicated.

Rx before an item indicates that a prescription must be obtained for its purchase. All other items may be purchased without a prescription through your pharmacy, many outfitters or the publisher.

BASIC KIT

Rx Cortisporin ophthalmic 1/8th ounce tube	1 to 3 tubes
Rx Phenergan tablets, 25 mg	10 to 30 tablets
Bisacodyl tablets, 5 mg	10 tablets
Rx Pontocaine ophthalmic .5% ointment, 1/8th oz. tube	1 tube
Camalox tablets	20 to 40 tablets
Rx Sumycin tablets, 250 mg - or E.E.S. 400 tablets	40 to 100 tablets
Rx Tylenol #3 tablets	10 to 30 tablets
Rx Actifed tablets	40 tablets
Povidone-iodine Prep Pads	10 pads
Bandages, 1" x 3" [plastic strips]	20 each
Gauze pads, 12 ply, 3" x 3" - sterile	20 each
Gauze roll, 3" x 10 yards, sterile	1 each
Elastic Bandage, 4" x 10 yards, top quality	1 each
Butterfly bandages, medium	10 each
Moleskin, 2" x 12" strip	1 each
Tape, 1" x 10 yards	1 roll

AUGMENTATION KIT

Rx Anakit, Hollister-Stier Co.	1 kit
Triple Antibiotic Ointment, 1½ gram packs	10 each
Hibiclens Surgical Scrub	2 to 4 ounces
Cutter Snake Bite Kit	1 kit
Vaseline Gauze, 3" x 9" - sterile	3 each
Needle Holder, Mayo-Hegar	1 each
Bandage Scissors, Lister, or Operating Scissors	1 only
Scalpel, Disposable, #10 or #11, sterile	1 only
Splinter Forceps	1 each
Ethilon Suture, 3-0	3 packs
Ethilon Suture, 5-0	3 packs
Plain Gut Suture, 3-0	1 pack
Tinactin Ointment 1%, 15 gram tube	1 tube
Rx Xylocaine for injection, 2% plain, 30 ml bottle	1 bottle
Rx Syringe, 3½ ml size with 25 gauge needle	2 each

A brief treatment outline guide and a relisting of the kit components has been printed on water resistant paper as the centerfold of this book for removal and inclusion in your medical kit. Full descriptions of the therapeutic application of the kit components are discussed under each medical subject in the text. A summary of the therapeutic uses of each item in the kit follows:

Rx CORTISPORIN OPHTHALMIC 1/8th ounce tube   1 to 3 tubes

A mixture of three antibiotics (polymyxin B, bacitracin and neomycin) and hydrocortisone (a steroid), this Burroughs-Wellcome product is primarily used in the eye for treatment of conjunctivitis due to bacterial infection. It is a versatile ointment which, in this book, is also used in the eye to treat allergic conjunctivitis and inflammation of the eye due to snow blindness and other causes, and as protection against infection when foreign bodies have been removed from the eye. It must not be used in the eye when the ulcers of herpes simplex are affecting the eye -- generally in this case, the lymph nodes in front of the ears are swollen and the patient has symptoms of the flu with very red conjunctiva (or whites) of the eyes. The versatility of this product is such that it can also be used to treat otitis externa(swimmer's ear) and as a topical ointment to prevent infection in cuts, abrasions and burns. It can also be used to treat poison ivy and other contact dermatitis problems. On long trips this ointment should be augmented with packets of triple antibiotic due to the cost of the small 1/8th ounce ophthalmic tubes. The neomycin component is a frequent skin sensitizer, so if a rash develops with use, or worsens, it must be discontinued. For eye use, apply three times daily; otherwise, apply two times a day.

Rx PHENERGAN TABLETS, 25 mg   10 to 30 tablets

This versatile product from Wyeth has many actions that are taken advantage of to augment other medications and reduce the number of drugs required in the medical kit. It is excellent against nausea and vomiting (1 tablet every 6 hours); it has antihistamine activity for allergic reactions (1 tablet every 6 hours); it augments pain medication allowing less narcotic to be used or to make it more effective (1 or 2 tablets every 6 hours, along with 1 or 2 Tylenol #3 every 4 hours); it acts as a sleeping medication (2 tablets at bedtime) and as an anti-anxiety agent (2 tablets every 6 hours as required). It is a phenothiazine, so it is best pregnant patients not take it routinely.

BISACODYL TABLETS, 5 mg   *10 tablets*

This laxative is very safe and effective. Normally, taking 1 or 2 tablets at bedtime will cause a bowel movement by morning. All laxatives can cause abdominal cramping, particularly in a constipated person. This is due to the increased motility of the gut caused by the laxative. Bisacodyl is virtually nontoxic.

Rx PONTOCAINE OPHTHALMIC, .5% ointment   *1 tube*
1/8th ounce tube

A sterile ointment made to relieve pain in the eye and to help in the removal of foreign bodies. This ointment will also relieve the pain of 1° burns and 2° burns. If a rash develops, its use must be discontinued. If the pain in the eye returns, a foreign body may be present and must be carefully excluded. This will also relieve the pain of swimmer's ear and sore gums from cold sores, etc.

CAMALOX TABLETS   *20 to 40 tablets*

A powerful antacid, this product by Rorer contains 200 mg of magnesium hydroxide, 225 mg of aluminum hydroxide and 250 mg calcium carbonate per tablet. Each tablet will neutralize 36 mEq of acid. Tablets are sealed in aluminum foil, ideal for field use, in strips of ten. Do not take this product with Sumycin, as it would prevent the Sumycin from working as well.

Rx SUMYCIN TABLETS, 250 mg   *40 to 100 tablets*

A tetracycline, this drug has a wide spectrum of activity and is frequently referred to throughout the text. These tablets made by Squibb will withstand rough usage and even damp conditions, unlike gelatine capsules. This drug should not be used by children under eight years of age or women in the last half of pregnancy. Dosage ranges from 1 tablet every 6 hours to 2 tablets every 4 hours.

In case of allergy to tetracycline (Sumycin), or if a youngster under age of eight or a woman in the last half of pregnancy must take an antibiotic, this item will have to be replaced in the basic Rx medical kit. I would advise using E.E.S. 400.

Rx E.E.S. 400   *40 to 100 tablets*

Erythromycin ethylsuccinate 400 mg. by Abbott is a firm tablet that resists abuse while on wilderness trips. It has a wide range of efficacy, but not as wide as tetracycline. Its use is discussed throughout the text. For a serious abdominal infection, such as appendicitis, it would pay to carry Cleocin 150 mg capsules (20 each) to be used instead of the EES 400. Cleocin and EES 400 should not be used at the same time as they are probably antagonistic and the two together would work less well than either separately. This is also true of tetracyclines (such as Sumycin) and penicillin, in case you intend carrying both of those types of drugs. Use them separately, not at the same time. EES 400 may be taken on either a full or empty stomach.

Rx TYLENOL #3   *10 to 30 tablets*

A mixture of 300 mg of acetaminophen and 30 mg of codeine phosphate, the principle use of this drug manufactured by McNeil Laboratories is the relief of pain. It will also lower temperature, stop a cough and help stop abdominal cramping and diarrhea. It will help with the treatment of itching, as itching is a type of pain stimulus. Dosage of 1 tablet every 4 to 6 hours should be adequate for a severe toothache, and we all know how bad those are. If necessary, 2 tablets every 4 hours could be taken for severe pain (see also the section on Phenergan).

Rx ACTIFED TABLETS   *40 tablets*

Each tablet contains 60 mg of pseudoephedrine (a vasoconstrictor) and 2.5 mg of triprolidine (an antihistamine). While these are available in Canada over the counter without a prescription, in the United States a prescription is required for purchase. The normal prescription usage is 1 tablet every 6 hours to relieve congestion in sinus and nasal passages due to virus and allergic problems. This product is mildly effective in asthma, but is not a drug of choice. It is excellent in opening the Eustachian tube for treatment and prevention of otitis media (middle ear infection or congestion). Note the section on pseudoephedrine listed in the Nonprescription (nonRx) Wilderness Expedition Medical Kit.

POVIDONE-IODINE PREP PADS   10 pads

Povidone-iodine is a virtually non-stinging, water soluable iodine complex which is non-staining to skin and natural fabrics. Non-irritating to skin and mucous membranes. It kills bacteria, fungi, viruses, protozoa and yeasts and has a more prolonged germicidal action than ordinary iodine solutions. It is more rapid in action than hexachlorophene. Useful in wiping surgical instruments, preparing wounds and cleaning the surgeon's hands. Pads are saturated, folded and sealed in individual use packets.

BANDAGE MATERIALS FOR THE BASIC KIT

Bandages, 1" x 3" [plastic strips]	20 each
Gauze pads, 12 ply, 3" x 3", sterile	20 each
Gauze roll, 3" x 10 yards, sterile	1 each
Elastic bandage, 4" x 10 yards, top quality	1 each
Butterfly bandages, medium	10 each
Moleskin, 2" x 12"	1 strip
Tape, 1" x 10 yards	1 roll

Obviously, the quantities of the above may have to be increased or decreased, depending upon the numbers of persons in the party, length of time in the field and risk of various injuries being encountered. But the above should handle most trips with a minimal amount of bulk and weight.

The following items should be considered as augmentation of the basic prescription wilderness expedition medical kit when weight permits:

Rx ANAKIT, Hollister-Stier   1 kit

For the treatment of anaphylactic shock of bee stings, etc. (see Page 91). This kit consists of 1 syringe containing 2 single doses epinephrine U.S.P. 1:1000 for subcutaneous injection; 4 tablets of chlorpheniramine 4 mg; 2 sterilizing swabs of 70% isopropyl alcohol, 1 tourniquet and 1 instruction booklet. Weight 1½ oz. Current retail cost from a pharmacy is about $8.00.

TRIPLE ANTIBIOTIC OINTMENT, 1½ gram foil packets   10 each

Each gram of this ointment contains bacitracin 400 units, neomycin sulfate 5 mg, and polymyxin B sulfate 5000 units. For use as a topical antibiotic in the prevention and treatment of minor *infections of abrasions and burns. A light coat is applied twice daily. This nonprescription product is not sold OTC for any other purpose. In an emergency, it can be used to combat otitis externa [swimmer's ear or outer ear infection], by applying some of the ointment to the outer part of the ear canal and allowing it to melt its way interiorly. It should not be used when there is a danger of a perforated ear drum, as neomycin in the middle ear may cause permanent deafness. This antibiotic combination is also only available for eye use with a prescription. The small tubes [1/8th ounce] dispensed for ophthalmic [eye] use are specially sterilized by the manufacturer. Again, the neomycin component is generally safe, but it is a skin sensitizer, which may make the eye inflammation worse. Triple antibiotic ointment is tricky stuff to use in the ear and eye and for that reason it should be left to a physician to prescribe in these areas. This ointment will not cure established soft tissue infections [abscess or cellulitis]. See page 83 for a discussion of handling these problems.*

HIBICLENS SURGICAL SCRUB   ½ to 4 ounces

This new product by Stuart [chlorhexidine gluconate 4%] far surpasses hexachlorophene and povidone-iodine scrub in its antiseptic action. Its duration and onset of action is much more impressive than either of those two products also. It is a nonprescription item, but it may be hard to find.

CUTTER SNAKE BITE KIT   1 each

Contains three, sized suction cups, scalpel, antiseptic, constriction band and instructions. Weight: 1 ounce. See page 93 in text for its use. Current cost is about $3.75.

VASELINE GAUZE, STERILE, 3" x 9"   3 each

For application to second and third degree burns, when treating by the closed method described in the text, see page 37. This sterile bandage is sealed in foil for transport.

NEEDLE HOLDER   1 each

The Mayo-Hegar needle holder, or equal, is necessary to hold the curved suture needle. See text, page 76, for information about its use.

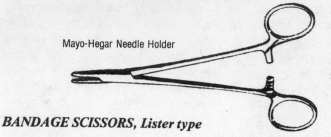

Mayo-Hegar Needle Holder

BANDAGE SCISSORS, Lister type   1 each

Bandage scissors have been designed to protect the patient with one blunt end and the other end not only blunt, but with a smooth, snag free knob to allow easy sliding under a tight bandage. These blunt ends also protect the carrying case from puncture while in storage. An alternate to the Lister bandage scissors would be the inclusion of operating scissors with two sharp points. These points can be protected with tape while in storage in the medical kit. They are useful for cutting tissue, nails and bandage material. Normally, a surgeon would not cut anything but tissue, as they would tend to be dulled by utilitarian work. However, the extra weight may not justify two sets of scissors in your medical kit.

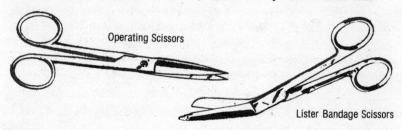

Operating Scissors

Lister Bandage Scissors

SCALPEL, DISPOSABLE, #10 or #11, STERILE   1 only

Used for a variety of surgical purposes, such as opening an abscess, these disposable units are sealed to preserve sterility until first used. By wiping with povidone-iodine prep pads, they could be resterilized for emergency use in the field.

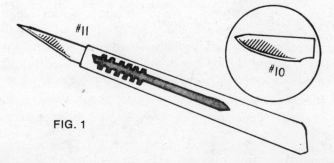

#11

#10

FIG. 1

SPLINTER FORCEPS   *1 each*

A sophisticated pair of tweezers, necessary to remove imbedded objects that one collides with so easily in the wilderness.

SUTURE, ETHILON 3-0 (heavy)   *3 packs*
SUTURE, ETHILON 5-0 (fine)   *3 packs*
SUTURE, PLAIN GUT 3-0   *1 pack*

For the surgical repair of wounds, see Pages 75-80 in the text. Package is sterile with attached curved needle. The 3-0 ethilon's needle is designated FS-1 for general repair use, while the 5-0 ethilon and 3-0 gut is supplied with an FS-2 needle. The FS-2 is a narrower gauge. The ethilon suture is a monofilament nylon, 18 inches in length. The plain gut suture is 27 inches long, packed in isopropyl alcohol within the foil packet.

TINACTIN OINTMENT, 15 gram tube   *1 tube*

Tinactin is the Schering brand name for a 1% tolnaftate cream, a very effective antifungal, that is highly successful in treating fungus infections of the skin which cause tinea pedis (athlete's foot), tinea cruris (jock itch) and tinea corporis (body ring worm). It is virtually nonsensitizing and does not ordinarily sting or irritate intact or broken skin. It is odorless and does not stain.

If you intend to suture with anesthesia to numb the skin, then you will require the following:

Rx XYLOCAINE for injection, 2%, 30 ml bottle   *1 each*
Rx SYRINGE - 3½ ml size with 25 gauge needle   *2 each*

It is easy to learn to use the above. Check with your physician and note the discussion on Pages 75 - 80 in the text.

Many other prescription drugs are mentioned in the text. If you have a high degree of suspicion that you may be encountering the problems mentioned where they are the drug of choice, then it may make sense to augment the kit with them.

All medications mentioned in the text are listed in the index starting on page 112.

THE NONPRESCRIPTION (nonRx) WILDERNESS
EXPEDITION MEDICAL KIT

The items listed in this kit are available "over the counter" (OTC) without prescription. The dosages and uses listed, however, do not necessarily conform to the OTC guidelines listed by the manufacturer, the FDA, or other agencies. Their use as indicated in this book should be restricted to healthy young adults not suffering from hypertension, diabetes, glaucoma, kidney disease, liver disease, thyroid disease or ladies who are pregnant or nursing their infants. Prior to embarking upon a wilderness expedition where such use of these items may be required, all participants should have a physical exam to insure their exclusion from the above categories.

This kit should be adequate for 2 to 10 persons on a trip into isolated areas lasting from 1 to 3 months. The BASIC KIT contains the essential items, while the AUGMENTATION KIT adds depth to the basic kit, notably the ability to suture lacerations and otherwise take care of trauma with more sophistication. It should be noted that while the needle holder and suture material are not prescription items, Xylocaine for numbing the skin and the syringe used to administrate it ARE! Thus, any suturing would have to be done without anesthesia, unless a prescription is obtained and those items carried.

The basic portion of the Nonprescription Wilderness Expedition Medical Kit can be used to treat nearly every emergency condition listed in this book. The total weight of the basic portion of this kit is 15½ ounces. The augmentation portion weighs an additional 9½ ounces. The total kit would thus weigh 25 ounces, using the largest number of the items indicated below.

All of the above items may be purchased without a prescription through your pharmacy, many outfitters or the publisher.

USE THERAPY INDICATED WITH EITHER THE Rx KIT OR THE nonRx KIT -- NOT FROM BOTH KITS AT THE SAME TIME.

BASIC KIT

Percogesic	24 to 48 tablets
Pseudoephedrine 30 mg	50 tablets
Chlorpheniramine 4 mg	25 tablets
Yellow Oxide of Mercury ophthalmic 1%, 1/8th oz tube	1 tube
Schein Otic Drops (or equal), 1 ounce bottle	1 bottle
Triple Antibiotic Ointment, 1½ ounce packets	10 packets
Dibucaine Ointment 1%, 15 gram tube	1 tube
Meclizine 25 mg tablets	10 tablets
Bacid Capsules	20 to 30 capsules
Bisacodyl tablets, 5 mg	10 tablets
Camalox tablets	20 to 40 tablets
Povidone-iodine Prep Pads	10 pads
Bandages, 1" x 3" [plastic strips]	20 each
Gauze pads, 12 ply, 3" x 3", sterile	20 each
Gauze roll, 3" x 10 yards, sterile	1 each
Elastic Bandage, 4" x 10 yards, top quality	1 each
Butterfly bandages, medium	10 each
Moleskin, 2" x 12" strip	1 each
Tape, 1" x 10 yards	1 roll

AUGMENTATION KIT

Vaseline Gauze, sterile, 3" x 9"	3 each
Hibiclens Surgical Scrub	½ to 4 ounces
Needle Holder, Mayo-Hegar	1 each
Bandage Scissors, Lister - or Operating Scissors	1 only
Scalpel, disposable, #10 or #11, sterile	1 only
Splinter Forceps	1 each
Ethilon Suture, 3-0	3 packs
Ethilon Suture, 5-0	3 packs
Plain Gut Suture, 3-0	1 pack
Cutter Snake Bite Kit	1 kit
Tinactin Ointment 1%, 15 gram tube	1 tube
Tooth Ache Gel, 1/8th ounce	1 tube

A brief treatment outline guide and a relisting of the kit components has been printed on water resistant paper as the centerfold of this book for removal and inclusion in your medical kit. Full description of the therapeutic application of the kit components are discussed under each medical subject in the text. A summary of the therapeutic uses of each item in the kit follows:

PERCOGESIC TABLETS   24 to 48 tablets

This, in my opinion, is the best pain medication and muscle relaxant available without a prescription. Each tablet contains acetaminophen 325 mg and phenyltoloxamine citrate 30 mg. The former is for pain and fever primarily, while the second component is a muscle relaxant and tranquilizer. Thus, this compound is particularly good for muscle sprains, tension headaches, minor orthopedic injuries, menstrual cramps, etc. It works well as a sedative when two are taken before bedtime. Just as other pain medications, it will help relieve itch. The normal dose for adults is two tablets every four hours, not to exceed 8 tablets in a day; for children 6 to 12 years, one half the adult dose. My recommended dosages for various problems are found throughout the text.

PSEUDOEPHEDRINE 30 mg TABLETS   50 tablets

Pseudoephedrine hydrochloride is a very effective vasoconstrictor and decongestant. It should be used for congestion, sneezing, runny nose, pressure of sinusitis and middle ear pressure of otitis media (middle ear infection) and mild asthma. The non-prescription instructions for taking this drug are one tablet three times daily. The same drug in a 60 mg tablet (twice the strength) combined with an antihistamine is available only by prescription in the United States, but is available in Canada OTC (without prescription). The normal dosage of the Rx drug in the U.S. is one tablet every 6 hours. In severe cases of head congestion, it would generally be appropriate to take two of the 30 mg tablets, along with a 4 mg chlorpheniramine, every 6 hours. Increased dosages are safe in virtually all people, but this use without consulting a physician should be avoided.

CHLORPHENIRAMINE 4 mg TABLETS   25 tablets

This is an antihistamine which is indicated to treat rhinitis (runny nose) due to allergy, conjunctivitis (eye irritation) due to inhaled allergy, allergic skin problems, and as an additional treatment adjunctive to epinephrine and other standard measures for anaphylactic shock due to snake bites, bee stings, and spider bites, after the acute manifestations have been controlled. The nonprescription dose is one tablet three to four times daily. This same compound in 8 mg capsules for every 12 hour use has been approved for OTC sale. However, 12 mg capsules still require an Rx in the United States.

YELLOW OXIDE OF MERCURY OPHTHALMIC 1%
1/8th ounce tube 1 tube

Before the advent of the prescription antibiotic eye medications, this was one of the best medications available for eye infection. The use of prescription antibiotics has eliminated the need to use this compound. Without treatment most bacterial conjunctivitis lasts only 10 to 14 days. This ointment may aid in speeding this recovery, but in the event of continued discomfort beyond the initial 3 to 4 days, or with ANY impairment of vision, a physician should be rapidly sought to prevent complications from unusual or severe infections which may possibly result in blindness.

SCHEIN OTIC DROPS 1 ounce bottle   1 bottle

A formulation of chloroxlenol, benzalkonium chloride, acetic acid, and glycerine. More than 90% of all external otitis (outer ear infection, swimmer's ear), can be treated with acetic acid in a vehicle such as glycerine. The other components of this preparation also provide antibacterial action. A preparation may not be sold over the counter with advertising claiming that it will cure these ear infections, it can only be sold to soften wax and to prevent them. In case of a severe otitis externa, a local antibiotic ointment will be needed. The triple antibiotic ointment, sold over the counter for minor skin laceration protection, is usable in this case, but this is not an indication for sale or an advertisable claim. A drop form of suspension works much better than the ointment as far as penetration is concerned. Very severe otitis externa will generally require oral antibiotics and perhaps even the use of steroids, but these are prescription drugs.

DIBUCAINE OINTMENT 1%, 15 gram tube   1 tube

This is a topical anesthetic which will very effectively anesthetize (numb) the skin for temporary relief of pain and itching associated with sunburn, minor burns, insect bites and stings, and hemorrhoids. For areas with broken skin, I would advise also applying triple antibiotic ointment.

MECLIZINE 25 mg TABLETS   10 tablets

Meclizine hydrochloride is a nonprescription drug, very useful in preventing motion sickness. The dosage is one tablet every 24 hours. Nausea and vomiting are very difficult to treat with nonprescription drugs, but this drug is exceptionally effective in prevent-

ing their occurrence due to motion. On a prescription basis only this drug is used to treat vertigo due to middle ear infection or other impairment. Under these conditions the use of the drug is increased to one tablet every 8 hours.

BACID CAPSULES, anti-diarrhea   20-30 capsules

Bacid capsules (Fisons Corporation) contain a specially cultured human strain of viable Lactobacillus acidophilus together with 100 mg of sodium carboxymethylcellulose per capsule. The idea is that the Lactobacillus, a bacteria, will replace the harmful bacteria causing the diarrhea. The carboxymethylcellulose absorbs fluids in the gut and acts as a vehicle for the storage of the powdered Lactobacillus. Although the latter is in a freeze-dried state, the manufacturer must recommend refrigeration of this product.

BISACODYL, 5 mg TABLETS   10 tablets

See description under the prescription medical kit listing.

CAMALOX TABLETS   20 to 40 tablets

See description under the prescription medical kit listing.

POVIDONE-IODINE PREP PADS   10 pads

See description under the presciption medical kit listing

BANDAGE MATERIALS FOR THE BASIC KIT

Bandages, 1" x 3" [Plastic strips]	*20 each*
Gauze pads, 12 ply, 3" x 3", sterile	*20 each*
Gauze roll, 3" x 10 yards, sterile	*1 each*
Elastic bandage, 4" x 10 yards, top quality	*1 each*
Butterfly bandages, medium	*10 each*
Moleskin, 2" x 12"	*1 strip*
Tape, 1" x 10 yards	*1 roll*

Obviously, the quantities of the above may have to be increased or decreased depending upon the numbers of persons in the party, length of time in the field, and risk of various injuries being encountered. But the above should handle most trips with a minimal amount of bulk and weight.

The following items should be considered as augmentation of the basic nonprescription wilderness expedition medical kit when weight permits:

Vaseline Gauze, sterile, 3" x 9"	*3 each*
Hibiclens surgical scrub	*¼ to 4 ounces*
Cutter Snake Bite Kit	*1 each*
Tinactin antifungal ointment, 15 grams	*1 tube*
Tooth Ache Gel, 1/8th ounce tube	*1 tube*
Needle Holder	*1 each*
Ethilon suture, 3-0	*3 each*
Ethilon suture, 5-0	*3 each*
Plain Gut Suture, 3-0	*1 each*
Bandage Scissors	*1 each*
Splinter forceps	*1 each*
Scalpel, disposable, #10 or #11, sterile	*1 only*

Descriptions of the above items may be found under the prescription medical kit listings with the exception of Tooth Ache Gel.

TOOTH ACHE GEL 1/8th ounce   1 tube

A gel comprised of benzocaine .5% and benzalkonium chloride in a special saliva resistant oral base, is ideal for tooth ache and sore gums from any cause -- a small bottle of oil of cloves (Eugenol) may be substituted for the tooth ache gel.

INCIDENTAL ITEMS USED BY THE TEAM MEDIC

Occasional use of items brought along for various other purposes is made for medical reasons. From the cook the medic needs to borrow baking soda, salt and sugar in the management of profound diarrhea. Soap for cleaning wounds may also be obtained from the kitchen, if a surgical scrub is not carried in the medical kit. Granulated sugar sprinkled on abrasions is a field expedient method of preventing infection, when there are no antibiotics available.

Each fishing kit should have wire cutters, possibly required to remove a hook from people, as well as fish. It may also be used to destroy a zipper if someone has caught their skin. Wool clothing is needed to prevent and treat hypothermic conditions, especially wool hat, wool socks and wool shirts. A tube tent may also be a useful emergency shelter for a wounded trip member, and helpful in preventing and treating hypothermia.

Matches are frequently a life-saver and should be available on each trip (note the other ten essentials on Page 1). And perhaps the entire party would benefit with a daily vitamin supplement, such as the formulation in the popular Miles Laboratories *One-A-Day with Iron*.

FEVER - CHILLS -- The average oral temperature of a resting individual is 98.6°F, and in active individuals 99.0°F. Rectal temperatures are 0.5 to 1°F higher. Temperature rise in a human will result in the heart rate increasing 10 beats per minute faster than the patient's normal resting temperature. This is a useful field method of judging temperature, if each individual knows what his resting pulse is. Some diseases cause a peculiar drop in heart rate even in the face of an obviously high temperature. The most notable of these is typhoid fever, pages 70 and 104.

Although injury and exposure can cause elevated body temperature, fever is usually the result of infection. The cause of the fever should be sought and treated. If pain or infection is located in the ear, throat, etc., refer to the appropriate anatomical area listed in the Instant Reference Clinical Index which starts on page 112.

If other symptoms beside fever are present (diarrhea, cough, etc.), see the cross references listing these symptoms in the Instant Reference Clinical Index in order to provide treatment to alleviate the suffering of these maladies. This may diagnose the underlying disease which would have a specific treatment indicated in the text.

The wilderness approach to therapy may be quite different from that used in clinical medicine. In the wilderness when in doubt about whether or not the fever is due to viral, bacterial, or other infectious causes - treat with antibiotic from your Rx medical kit. Initially, give the patient Sumycin, 250 mg., two tablets every six hours and continue until the fever has broken, then reduce the dose to one tablet every six hours for an additional four days. If it is possible that the patient has a strep throat (see page 33), make sure to provide antibiotic coverage for ten days. If Rocky Mountain Spotted Fever is a possibility, (see page 74), continue coverage for a total of 14 days. If you are not carrying the Rx kit, then treat the symptoms using the medications described in your nonRx kit. In either case, rest is important until the patient is again free of fever and has a sense of well being.

Chills are a state of shivering with a sense of coldness - not related to hypothermia as discussed on pages 52 to 54. Chills are usually followed by fever. They frequently indicate the onset of a bacterial infection which should be treated with an antibiotic as described above.

SHOCK -- THIS IS A LIFE THREATENING EMERGENCY and must be treated promptly. Insure that an adequate airway is established. (Note further discussion under ARTIFICIAL RESPIRATION, Page 41). Assess cardiac status -- place hand over a carotid artery, located in the upper neck along side of the trachea (windpipe). In shock the patient will have a weak, rapid pulse -- in adults the rate will be over 140, children over 180 beats per minute. If there is doubt about a pulse being present, listen to the bare chest -- if cardiac standstill is present, institute cardio-pulmonary resusitation (see discussion under CARDIAC COMPRESSION, Page 42). Elevate the legs to 45° to obtain a rapid return of venous blood to the heart -- however, if there has been a head injury, lay the patient flat. If external bleeding is evident, stop with direct pressure (use a bare hand, if necessary until an adequate bandage can be obtained or fashioned). Attempt to treat the underlying cause of the shock -- a quick history may well elicit the cause of the shock and appropriate treatment can be devised from the field expedient methods listed in this book.

An important aspect of the correction of shock is to identify and treat the underlying cause. Shock can be caused by burns, electrocution, hypothermia, bites, stings, bleeding, fractures, pain, hyperthermia, high altitude cerebral edema, profound diarrhea, illness, rough handling, just to name a few. Obviously, at times the history of the patient's past 24 hours is helpful in making the correct diagnosis -- most frequently a quick glance is enough to tell the tale. Each of these underlying causes is discussed separately in the text.

PAIN -- Adequate pain management can be a mixture of proper medication and attitude -- the attitude of both the victim and the medic being important. A calm, professional approach to problems will lessen anxiety, panic and pain. From the nonRx kit provide the victim with Percogesic, 1 or 2 tablets every 4 hours. Percogesic (made by Endo Laboratories) is probably the best pain medication that can be obtained without a prescription. Each tablet contains 325 mg of acetaminophen and 30 mg of phenyltoloxamine citrate. The latter is a muscle relaxant, which makes this a particularly good medication for orthopedic injuries or whenever muscle sprains and contusions are encountered. It is also ideal for menstrual cramps, tension headache, and it is relatively safe to use in head injuries. It contains no aspirin, so it would not tend to enhance any internal bleeding in a head injury. It can also be used for the muscle ache and fever from viral and bacterial infections.

Aspirin has anti-inflammatory capabilities that acetaminophen (Tylenol) does not. For a tendonitis, bursitis, or arthritic pain, aspirin is generally a better choice. Avoid the use of aspirin in gouty arthritis, as it may make the condition worse. It should also not be used by many asthmatics. The ideal aspirin product for wilderness use is the 5 grain enteric coated tablet. These hard coated tablets will not disintegrate with rough handling and high humidity conditions. Dosage would generally be 1 or 2 tablets every 4 hours. Both aspirin and percogesic are ideal in the treatment of itch! The itch sensation is transmitted along pain nerve fibers, so that these analgesic medications specifically aid in its management. FOR SEVERE PAIN, you may have to rely on the prescription medical kit, and take 1 or 2 Tylenol #3 every 4 hours. Each tablet contains 300 mg acetaminophen and 30 mg of codeine phosphate. One of these tablets is generally enough to eliminate a bad toothache. For serious injury, 2 tablets at a time provide fairly substantial relief. They can be augmented by also giving the victim one 25 mg Phenergan tablet every 4 to 6 hours. This medication helps eliminate the nausea associated with high codeine dosages, and from my experience it potentiates the narcotic so that it works much better.

EYE PROBLEMS

Pain and irritation of the eye can be devastating. Causes are listed on the table below:

CAUSES OF EYE PAIN

FOREIGN BODY - p.23
INFECTION - BACTERIAL - p.25
         VIRAL - p.25
         STYE - p.26
ALLERGIC - p.27
ABRASION - COLD TEMPERATURE - p.24
         WIND - p.24
         MECHANICAL - p.24
SNOW BLINDNESS - p.25
STRAIN - p.26
GLAUCOMA - p.26

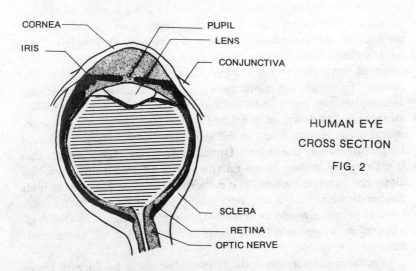

HUMAN EYE
CROSS SECTION
FIG. 2

The most common problems in the wilderness will be foreign body, abrasion, and infection (conjunctivitis). Therapy for these problems is virtually the same, except that it is very important to remove any foreign body that may be present.

The initial step in examining the painful eye is to remove the pain. One of the lessons drilled into us in medical school was to never, *never* write a prescription for eye anesthesia agents (such as Pontocaine .5% which I recommend taking along in the wilderness medical kit). The reason is that the patient may use it and then not have his eye carefully examined for a foreign body. Eventually, this foreign body may cause an ulcer to form in the cornea doing profound damage. So when using the Pontocaine, remember, it is very important to insure that no such foreign body exists. Pull down on the lower lid and instill a thin ribbon of the Pontocaine ophthalmic ointment. Have the patient close his eye and let him rest with it shut, thus giving time for the medication to melt and anesthetize the eye. This medication burns when initially used.

After the patient has calmed down, have him open the eye and look straight ahead. Very carefully shine a pen light at the cornea from one side to see if a minute speck becomes visable. By moving the light back and forth, one might see movement of a shadow on the iris of the eye, and thus confirm the presence of a foreign body. The Pontocaine ointment will give a gooey appearance to the cornea that may mimic a foreign body. Have the victim blink to move any medication around. A point that consistently stays put with blinking is probably a foreign body. Take a sterile, or at least a clean, Q-tip and approach the foreign body from the side. Gently prod it with the Q-tip handle until it is loosened. Frequently it will stick to the handle. Otherwise use the cotton portion to touch it for removal once the foreign body has been dislodged from the cornea. Of course, a stoic patient could undergo this without Pontocaine, but using anesthesia makes the patient more comfortable and cuts down on the blink reflex (interference). After removal of the foreign body, instill some antibiotic. The prescription kit should contain Cortisporin Ophthalmic 1/8 oz. tube. Again, this is instilled by pulling down on the lower lid and laying a ribbon along the everted margin. Have the patient close his eye to melt the medication. About the best non-prescription eye medication for this purpose would be Yellow Oxide of Mercury 1% Ophthalmic Ointment, also in a 1/8 oz. tube and instilled in the same manner.

In making the foreign body examination, also be sure to check under the eyelids. Evert the upper lid over a Q-tip stick, thus examining not only the eyeball, but also the undersurface of the eyelid. This surface may be gently brushed with the cotton applicator to eliminate minute particles. Always use a fresh Q-tip when touching the eye or eyelid an additional time.

EYE ABRASION -- The abrasion may be caused by a glancing blow from a wood chip, from a branch, or even from blowing ice and snow. The involved eye should be anesthetized with Pontocaine and protected with the Cortisporin ophthalmic ointment or yellow oxide of mercury as mentioned above. Make sure that no foreign body is still present. In cold wind, be sure to protect your eye from the effects of both blowing particles of ice and the wind itself. Grey Owl, in his interesting book, *TALES OF AN EMPTY CABIN*, tells how he was hiking on one of his long trips through the backwoods along a windswept frozen lake, when suddenly he lost all vision of the tree line. He felt that he must be in a white-out, so he turned perpendicular to the wind and hiked to shore. Suddenly he bumped into a tree and then realized that he was blind! He saved himself only by digging a snow cave and staying put for three days. He wondered how many good woodsmen were lost on their trap lines by such a similar incident, apparently an abrasion or temporary freezing of the cornea.

SNOW BLINDNESS -- This severely painful condition is caused by ultraviolet rays of the sun, which are considerably reflected by snow, water and sand. Thin cloud layers allow the transmission of these rays, while holding back the infra-red (heat) rays of the sun. Thus, it is possible on a rather cool, overcast day under bright snow conditions to become snow blind. Obviously, sunglasses are the preventative measure, or eliminating the glare by making slit glasses from any material at hand -- to include the ubiquitous bandanna. The ideal treatment is the use of Pontocaine ophthalmic to ease the pain. Cortisporin ophthalmic ointment may be used to decrease the inflammatory reaction and prevent infection or, from the non-prescription kit, give Percogesic 2 tablets every 4 hours for pain, and yellow oxide of mercury ophthalmic ointment to prevent infection. Patch the eyes to allow rest.

INFECTION -- An infection of the eye will be heralded by a scratchy feeling, almost indistinguishable from a foreign body being in the eye. The sclera or white of the eye will be reddened. Generally the eye will be mattered shut in the morning with pus or granular matter. Cortisporin ophthalmic ointment should be instilled three times a day for 5 to 7 days, certainly until all evidence of the infection has cleared. Steroids should not be placed in the eye if there is any chance that a viral infection may then cause corneal ulceration. The non-prescription kit should best carry the yellow oxide of mercury ophthalmic 1%. Instill this three times a day if the nonRx kit is being used.

If the redness persists longer than three days, the antibiotic may not be proper for the infection; in fact, the eye may be sensitive to it and it may actually be causing harm. Certainly stop its use and switch to another, such as Garamycin Ophthalmic. Professional assistance is needed immediately in cases of severe eye infections which are indicated by: the pupil becoming fixed and not reacting to light; the cornea of the pupil becoming cloudy; the iris around the pupil becoming irregular and not a perfect circle; or the white of the eye being very red around the iris and less red further away. (Simple pink eye or common conjunctivitis will generally be reddened over the surface of the white of the eye, but somewhat whiter next to the iris.) Although these severe infections of the eye are quite rare, they are a medical emergency that must be treated by a physician or blindness may result. Immediately start the patient on oral antibiotic (Rx Sumycin 250 mg. 4x daily), treat for pain (Rx Tylenol No. 3 or non-Rx Percogesic, one or two tablets every 4 hours), and evacuate, or blindness may result. Incidentally, simple pink eye or conjunctivitis will generally heal without medication in 10 to 14 days.

GLAUCOMA -- Glaucoma is the rise of pressure within the eyeball. The most common form (open angle glaucoma) generally is not encountered before the age of 40, with increasing frequency thereafter. The patient notes halos around lights, mild headaches, loss of vision to the sides (peripheral field cuts), and loss of ability to see well at night. This frequently affects both eyes. This is generally of gradual onset, so that the patient may consult a physician upon his return from the bush. The external eye usually appears normal. Initial treatment is with a prescription drug, one drop of 0.5% Pilocarpine. This malady should be detected by the pre-trip physical examination. Everyone over the age of 40 should have his intraocular pressure tested prior to departure. In fact, this should be checked yearly, regardless, in this age group.

STRAIN -- Strain is also characterized by headaches and some blurring of vision. This problem can become severe if glasses are lost early on a trip. Always carry a second pair of eyeglasses if you have prescription lenses. A pair of prescription sunglasses do not count as the second pair. I have been on several long trips where someone has suffered grievously because of this oversight.

A simple eye chart examination is not always sufficient to detect eye strain. An ophthalmologist or optometrist must perform refraction studies to determine visual acuity.

STIES AND CHALAZIA -- These infections of the eyelid can cause scratching of the cornea surface. Often the victim thinks that he has something in his eye when, in fact, one of these small pimples is forming. The sty is an infection along a hair follicle on the eyelid margin. The Chalazion is an infection of an oil gland on the inner lid margin. The eye should be protected with (Rx) Cortisporin ophthalmic or (nonRx) yellow oxide of mercury ophthalmic, applied three times daily. The sty may be carefully opened with a #11 scalpel blade and the pus wiped away with the edge of a gauze pad. if an oral antibiotic is available, it may also be taken until the condition resolves, (Rx) Sumycin, 250 mg four times daily. Wet hot packs should be applied for 15 minutes four times a day to draw the infection to a head.

SPONTANEOUS SUBCONJUNCTIVAL HEMORRHAGE -- This is mentioned only to tell you not to worry about it. This not-infrequent problem comes from a rupture of a small blood vessel in the sclera or white of the eye. There is no pain associated with this problem. The patient is generally told by someone else that their eye is bright red, or they notice it in the mirror. The hemorrhage will turn the involved portion of the eye bright red. This takes several weeks to totally disappear, but no therapy is required. This condition can occur with other symptoms in people afflicted by trichinosis (see Page 64).

BLUNT TRAUMA TO THE EYE -- The immediate treatment is to immobilize the injured eye as soon as possible by patching both eyes and moving the patient only by litter. Double vision means that there has been a fracture of the orbit of the eye or that there is a lesion within the central nervous system. Double vision is sometimes caused by swelling of tissue behind the eyelid. A puncture wound or foreign bodies should be treated by a physician. Start the patient on an oral antibiotic (Rx Sumycin 250 mg 4x daily), and provide the strongest pain medication necessary to prevent the patient squeezing his eye and thus injuring intraocular contents even more. Frankly, small corneal or scleral lacerations may require no treatment at all. But severe injury to one eye may even cause blindness to develop in the other eye due to sympathetic ophthalmia which is probably an allergic response to eye pigment of the injured eye entering the victim's blood stream.

ALLERGIC CONJUNCTIVITIS -- The common wilderness causes are sensitivity to inhaled pollens and irritation with wood smoke. This problem is usually associated with a runny nose (rhinitis) and at times swelling of the eyelids, the appearance of welts (urticaria) and severe itching. In severe cases, there may even be considerable swelling of the conjunctival covering of the white of the eye, forming what appears as fluid-filled sacs over the sclera of the eye (but not covering the cornea). Treatment with the prescription kit would include application of the Cortisporin ophthalmic ointment every four hours and giving a compound with antihistamine action such as Phenergan, 25 mg 4 times daily for the duration of the problem. Or, from the nonRx kit, give the chlorpheniramine 4 mg, one tablet every six hours and medication for pain such as Percogesic, one or two tablets every six hours. Use therapy indicated with either the Rx kit or the nonRx kit -- not from both kits at the same time.

NOSE CONGESTION -- is caused by allergic reaction to pollen, dust, or other allergens, viral upper respiratory infections, or bacterial respiratory infections. Bacterial infections will require an antibiotic to cure, but otherwise all three are treated similarly for symptomatic relief. The runny nose can be cleared up with the use of the oral vasoconstrictor pseudoephedrine and an antihistamine which specifically help with allergic problems, but which also provide a drying action for all three problems. From the nonprescription kit place the patient on pseudoephedrine (brand name Sudafed), 30 mg tablets. The OTC instructions are one every eight hours. Generally it will be necessary to use two every six hours to obtain relief. The addition of an OTC antihistamine chlorpheniramine 4 mg every four hours will also be helpful (brand name Chlortrimeton). In the U.S. a prescription product consisting of pseudoephedrine, 60 mg and an antihistamine which is ideal for this use is Actifed, taken every six hours. This product is available without a prescription in Canada. If the patient has no elevation in temperature, don't bother giving him an antibiotic. A low grade temp is probably viral and still does not warrant an antibiotic, as it will not kill or in any way harm a virus.

Enlarged lymph glands may mean either a viral or bacteria infection. A tender gland, one that hurts when touched, generally means the infection is bacterial and that an antibiotic should be provided. The antibiotics included in the Wilderness Prescription Medical Kit should be very helpful, namely (Rx) Sumycin, 250 mg four times daily, or the alternative (Rx) EES 400, 4 times daily. The body will generally eliminate the infection on its own even without antibiotics.

SINUS CONGESTION AND HEADACHE are treated as above, generally with the use of the antibiotic, if available, and the addition of pain medication, (non Rx) Percogesic, one or two tablets every four hours being ideal.

NOSE BLEED -- is generally from small arteries in the front of the nose partition or nasal septum. The best treatment is direct pressure. Have the victim squeeze the nose between his fingers for ten minutes by the clock (a very long time when there is no clock to watch). If this fails, squeeze another ten minutes. Do not blow the nose for this will dislodge clots and start the bleeding all over again. Give the victim a nasal decongestant such as pseudoephedrine, two 30 mg tablets 4 times a day and an antihistamine such as chlorpheneramine, 4 mg four times a day to help prevent sneezing and decrease nasal blood flow. Or, from the Rx kit, give Actifed, 1 tablet 4 times a day, rather than the pseudoephedrine and chlorpheneramine. Nose bleeds from fractures and blows to the nose are generally self-limited and will soon stop. Cold compresses to the back of the neck and forehead are of little help, but are better than nothing in severe cases of posterior nose bleed. Have the victim sit up to prevent choking on blood and to aid in reduction of the pressure of the nasal blood flow. After the bleeding has been controlled, have the victim place white petroleum jelly (Vaseline) in the septum for several days to prevent further drying effect of breathing and hopefully prevent further bleeding.

NOSE FRACTURE -- As mentioned, the nose bleed associated with this will generally stop with pressure at the end of the nose. If the nose is laterally displaced or shoved to one side, push it back into place. More of these fractures have been treated by coaches on the playing field than have been reduced by doctors. If it is a depressed fracture, a specialist will have to properly elevate the fragments. Stabilize with a segment of aluminum finger splint, if available. Otherwise this is not necessary. As soon as the victim returns from the bush, have him seen by a physician, but this is not a reason for expensive medical evacuation. The best pain medication for nasal pain would be (Rx) Tylenol No. 3 or, (nonRx) Percogesic. Avoid the use of aspirin products as they tend to promote bleeding.

EAR PAIN SUMMARY

SOURCE OUTSIDE THE EAR
 DENTAL PAIN OR ABSCESS - p.34
 SORE THROAT OR LYMPH NODE - p.33
OUTER EAR INFECTION (SWIMMER'S EAR,
  OTITIS EXTERNA) - p. 30
MIDDLE EAR INFECTION (OTITIS MEDIA) - p.31

EARACHE -- Pain in the ear is either due to an infection behind the tympanic membrane (eardrum), in the outer ear canal, or due to infection elsewhere (generally a toothache, infected tonsil, or lymph node in the neck near the ear). The definitive method of examining the ear is to use the otoscope, an instrument with a light that allows ready visualization of the outer ear canal and of the ear drum. This device is expensive and requires training in use -- certainly it is not needed on wilderness expeditions. In the bush a simple physical exam will readily (and generally accurately) tell the etiology of the ear pain. A swollen tender nodule in the neck near the ear would be an *infected lymph node*. *Dental caries*, or *cavities*, can be identified by an exam of the mouth. If an obvious cavity is not present with visualization using a pen light or flashlight, try tapping on each tooth to see if pain is suddenly elicited. (See DENTAL PAIN).

Similarly, an abscess originating from the teeth will cause pain upon tapping the tooth in question and will generally show some swelling of the alveolar ridge, or gums, near the affected tooth. (See DENTAL ABSCESS.)

Most people with an earache have very accurately localized the source of the pain to the ear. The main question is whether it is middle ear pain from behind the eardrum, or an external auditory canal infection.

OUTER EAR INFECTION -- The external auditory meatus (or ear canal) generally gets inflamed due to swimmer's ear. This is officially called *external otitis*. Without a light one can determine if this is the case by pushing on the nob in front of the ear canal called the tragus. If this causes pain, then it is usually an external infection. This should be treated with ear drops containing antibiotic and an anti-inflammatory agent. These are only available with a prescription. I generally use Cortisporin otic, 4 drops every 3 to 4 hours. Wet a small piece of cotton with the solution and place in the ear canal to hold the medication in place. For wilderness trips I prefer to use the Cortisporin ophthalmic ointment. It has a different vehicle which is very gentle on the eye, but usable in the ear. The ear drops should never be used in the eye as they would cause considerable irritation. This helps cut down on the medications needed in the medical kit.

Severe infections will also need pain medication (Rx) Tylenol #3, 1 tablet every 4 hours; or (nonRx) Percogesic, 2 tablets every 4 hours. Severe infection will also need an oral antibiotic (Rx) Sumycin 250 mg 1 tablet every 6 hours.

To prevent external otitis, there are several non-prescription preparations (Schein Otic; Aquaear (Miller and Morton); Aurinol (National); Aqua-Otic-B (Ortega); Debrox drops (International); Stall Otic Drops (Cencil); Columbia Ear Drops (Columbia Medical)). These preparations use mixtures of boric acid, propylene glycol, glycerine, acetic acid, benzalkonium chloride and other ingredients to eliminate water, wax and bacteria. They are not as effective in treating a full-blown infection as the prescription products which contain various antibiotics and anti-inflammatory agents (steroids), but they are valuable in preventing it. If no prescription drugs are available, their use is better than nothing.

The external ear infection is frequently found to be due to high humidity conditions and wax accumulation, which these drops help neutralize. Triple antibiotic ointment can be gently applied with a Q-tip.

MIDDLE EAR INFECTION -- The *middle ear infection* will not be helped with ear drops. It has its origin in the accumulation of fluid behind the eardrum. This is usually prevented by the Eustachian tube, or auditory tube, which connects the middle ear to the throat and provides equalization of air pressure and subsequently prevents a vacuum from pulling fluid into the middle ear. The Eustachian tube can be blocked in any condition that would lead to a runny nose (rhinitis). Bacterial, viral, even allergic conditions can thus lead to the formation of fluid in the inner ear. This in itself will be painful and may not mean that an infection is present. The symptoms will generally be pain and hearing loss on the affected side(s). The patient will frequently say that if he could only yawn and pop his ear, it would feel better.

Regardless of the cause of the fluid build-up, several medications are nonprescription items. First, a vasoconstrictor is very helpful in shrinking the blood engorged membranes of the head and hopefully allowing the Eustachian tube to become functional again and promote the internal drainage/absorption of the fluid behind the eardrum. In the U.S., the best nonprescription drug for this purpose is pseudoephedrine 30 mg (one brand name is Sudafed). The over-the-counter instructions are to take this medication 1 tablet three times daily for an adult. The same medication in a 60 mg tablet is a prescription-only product in the U.S. In Canada it can be obtained OTC. The normal prescription dosage is one 60 mg tablet four times a day (every 6 hours).

The addition of an antihistamine is also indicated. A good over-the-counter preparation is chlorpheneramine (one brand name is ChlorTrimeton) 4 mg. In amounts larger than 4 mg, this also is a prescription-only product. The OTC instructions for this drug (4 mg size) are 1 tablet every 4 to 6 hours -- this should be an adequate dose, especially when coupled with the pseudoephedrine taken 60 mg every 6 hours. A combination product, Actifed, is a mixture of 60 mg of pseudoephedrine and an antihistamine -- available only by prescription in the U.S.; it is an OTC item in Canada.

The above regimen will cure the otitis media problem (middle ear infection) due to viral and allergic causes. If bacterial involvement of the middle ear fluid becomes a problem, the patient will need to be on a prescription antibiotic. The drug of choice differs by age group (due to prevalent bacteria in certain age groups). For the young adult making wilderness trips, the main antibiotic of this book, Sumycin 250 mg every 6 hours, or its alternative EES 400 every 6 hours, should handle the problem. A purulent (pus, i.e. bacterial) otitis media may cure itself by suddenly rupturing the eardrum and then easily draining to the outside. A sudden decrease in pain will occur. Hearing has already been decreased by the fluid accumulated behind the eardrum. This ruptured tympanic membrane (eardrum), generally heals very well. This should be treated by a physician upon return to civilization, but if the patient is being treated with antibiotics, this is not an indication to abort the trip.

SORE THROAT -- The common cause of a sore throat is viral pharyngitis. While uncomfortable, this malady requires no antibiotic treatment -- in fact, the antibiotic will do no good whatsoever. Strictly speaking, the sore throat that needs to be treated is the one caused by a specific bacteria (one of the streptococcus bacteria), as it has been found that treatment for ten days will avoid the dreaded complication of rheumatic fever which may occur in 1% to 3% of the people with this particular infection. Many purists in the medical profession feel that no antibiotics should be used until the results of a throat culture proving strep throat have returned from the lab (generally a two to three day wait). On a short trip, the victim can be taken to a doctor for a strep plate (throat culture) to determine if the sore throat was indeed strep. On a wilderness trip longer than one week, it would be best to commit the patient to a ten day therapy of antibiotic, realizing that he will soon be well -- but that it is essential to continue the medication for ten days. There are text book differences in the general appearance of a viral and bacterial sore throat -- the lymph nodes (or glands) in the neck are swollen in both cases, but they are very tender in bacterial infections; the throat will be quite red in bacterial infection; a white splotchy coating over the red tonsils or posterior throat generally means a bacterial infection -- at least, these classic indications are present 20% of the time. However, in young adults sore throats caused by virus (mononucleosis and adenovirus), may mimic all of the above. While the ideal antibiotic for strep throat is penicillin, from the Wilderness Prescription Medical Kit recommended in this book, you will have to use (Rx) Sumycin 250 mg 4 times daily for 10 days.

INFECTIOUS MONONUCLEOSIS -- A disease of young adults (teens through 30 years of age), generally presents as a terrible sore throat, swollen lymph nodes (normally posterior neck and not as tender as with bacterial infection), and a profound tired feeling. This disease is self-limited with total recovery to be expected after two weeks for most victims -- some, unfortunately are bed-ridden up to six months. Spleen enlargement is common -- the most serious aspect of this disease is the possibility of splenic rupture -- but this is rare. Avoid palpating the spleen (i.e. shoving on the left upper quadrant of the stomach) -- let the victim *rest* -- no hiking, etc. until the illness and feeling of lethargy has passed. The first five days are the worst. Give Percogesic for pain and temperature from the nonRx kit or, Tylenol #3 may be given every 4 to 6 hours from the Rx kit. For severe throat or ear pain, commit the patient to antibiotics for 10 days, as there will be no way of proving the diagnosis of mononucleosis in the wilderness. You may think you are dealing with mono, but actually have a strep pharyngitis. Both are mildly contagious. A mild form of hepatitis may occur with mononucleosis that requires no specific treatment other than rest.

DENTAL PAIN -- Cavities may be identified by visual examination of the mouth in most cases. At times, the pain is so severe that the patient cannot tell exactly which tooth is the offender. In that case, tap each tooth in turn until the offending one is reached -- a tap on it will elicit strong pain. Dry the tooth and try to clean out any cavity found. Apply (nonRx) Tooth Ache Gel, or eugenol to the cavity to aid in direct relief. (Rx) Tylenol #3 will generally eliminate the most severe dental pain -- (nonRx) use Percogesic. If an antibiotic is available, start the patient on (Rx) Sumycin 250 mg, 1 tablet 4 times daily or (Rx) EES 400 4 times daily.

DENTAL ABSCESS -- This consists of swelling of the gum under the tooth, sometimes the entire jaw may become swollen. This should be treated with an antibiotic and pain medication as above.

GINGIVITIS -- Or infection/inflammation of the gums should be treated with an antibiotic such as the (Rx) Sumycin 250 mg 4 times daily or EES 400 4 times daily. Rinse the mouth every two hours with salt water, if possible. Swish this water between teeth to loosen food particles. After a few days, when the inflammation has calmed down, start brushing and using dental floss, which should be in every personal kit, along with the tooth brush.

LOST FILLING -- This could turn into a real disaster. A lost filling replacement kit, for wilderness use, can be purchased from the publisher of this book. It consists of zinc oxide powder (not the ointment) and eugenol. Dry the cavity bed thoroughly with a gauze square. Place several drops of eugenol on the cavity to deaden the pain. Mix the zinc oxide powder with eugenol in about equal parts until a putty is formed. This always takes considerable more zinc oxide powder than at first would seem necessary. Pack this putty into the cavity and allow to set over the next 24 hours. Obviously avoid biting on this side. See a dentist as soon as possible as the loss of the filling may mean that extension of the cavity or weakening of the tooth structure has occurred.

MOUTH BLISTERS -- Frequently "cold sores" will develop with fever or with simple exposure to sunlight. They are especially prone to develop under stressful conditions. Antibiotics will be of no help, but if a secondary infection appears to have developed, use the (Rx) Sumycin 250 mg four times daily or (Rx) EES 400 four times daily. The direct application of toothache gel, or eugenol may be of some help. The toothache gels consisting of benzocain and benzalkonium chloride have been formulated with a special base to help prevent their easily washing away in the saliva. An interesting remedy would be the use of the bacid capsule, described elsewhere under treatment of diarrhea. For some reason the Lactobacillus acidophilus bacteria, which are in these capsules in a freeze-dried form, have been felt by many to promote the healing of cold sores. The capsule may be opened and the powdered content sprinkled directly upon the lesion.

The antibiotic regimen may work, based upon the repeated isolation of alpha-hemolytic streptococcus from these lesions. Their total duration untreated is 10 to 14 days.

SPRAIN -- Unusual stress across a joint can result in damage to supporting ligaments. Ordinarily this is a temporary stretching damage, but in severe cases, rupture of ligaments can result. These injuries must be "rested out", not "worked out"! A torn ligament is a serious problem and may require surgical repair - this is best done immediately, but can be safely delayed 2 to 3 weeks. Proper care of stretched ligaments must be started immediately. Whether stretched or torn, or even fractured - optimun care is avoiding any effort that causes increased pain at the involved joint (ankle, knee, wrist, elbow, etc.). Stretched ligaments will repair themselves and actually tighten up somewhat, but this is impossible if too much additional stress is applied.

Treatment of sprains, regardless of severity, is as follows: 1) apply cold for the first two days - as continuously as possible. Afterward, applying heat for 20 minutes, four times daily is helpful. Cold decreases the circulation, which lessens bleeding ans swelling. Heat increases circulation, which then aids the healing process. This technique applies to all injuries -- including muscle contusions. 2) Elevate the involved joint, if possible. 3) Wrap with elastic bandage or cloth tape to immobilize the joint and provide moderate support once ambulation (use) begins. Take care that wrappings are not so tightly applied that they cut off circulation. 4) Use crutches or other support to take enough weight off an injured ankle or knee to the point that increased pain is not experienced. The patient should not use an injured joint if such use causes pain, as this causes further stress on the already stressed ligaments or fracture. Conversely, if use of the injured part does not cause pain, additional damage is not being done. 5) If the victim must walk on an injured ankle or knee, and doing so causes considerable pain, then support it the best way possible (wrapping, crutches, tight boot for ankle injury, decreased carrying load) and realize that further damage is being done, but that in your opinion the situation warrants such a sacrifice. Under emergency movement conditions, a boot should not be removed from an injured ankle, as it may be impossible to get it back on. However, one must avoid too much compression of the soft tissue swelling to prevent circulation impairment. Doing considerable additional damage to the ankle and risking circulation damage to the rest of the foot is an important decision to make. 6) Treat for pain - from the Rx kit use Tylenol #3, one tablet every four hours as needed, or from the nonRx kit use Percogesic, one or two tablets every four hours. See also the discussion of fractures on pages 86 - 89.

BURNS -- Most important in the management of burns is the severity of the lesion (degree) and the amount of surface involved. *Figure 3* depicts the Rule of Nines in determining the percent of body involvement. An entire arm equals 9%, therefore the burn of one side of just the forearm would equal 2%. The chest and back equal 18% and the abdomen and back equal 18%. The proportions are slightly different for children.

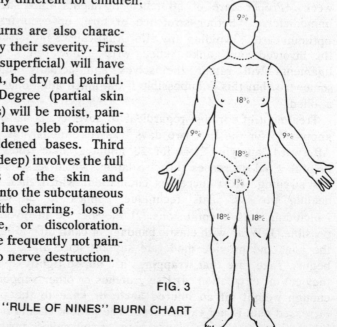

Burns are also characterized by their severity. First Degree (superficial) will have erythema, be dry and painful. Second Degree (partial skin thickness) will be moist, painful, and have bleb formation with reddened bases. Third Degree (deep) involves the full thickness of the skin and extends into the subcutaneous tissue with charring, loss of substance, or discoloration. These are frequently not painful due to nerve destruction.

FIG. 3

"RULE OF NINES" BURN CHART

TREATMENT OF BURNS depends upon the extent and severity of the lesion. As soon as possible remove the source of burn -- quick immersion into cool water will help eliminate additional heat from scalds or burning fuels and clothing. Or otherwise suffocate the flames with clothing, sand, etc. Running will fan flames and increase the injury.

A. *FIRST AND SECOND DEGREE BURNS INVOLVING LESS THAN 15% OF AN ADULT (10% OF CHILD)* -- Cleanse the area with nonmedicated soap and water and rinse thoroughly. All grease and foreign material should be removed. Large blisters may be lanced and the collapsed skin allowed to cover the wound. Apply a sterile vaseline gauze dressing, or, in first degree burns, 1% dibucaine ointment (which should result in almost complete pain relief). This dressing should be changed in a maximum of 3 days, preferably every 48 hours. First degree burns will have healed in that time and require no further treatment.

Immobilize and elevate burned extremities, if possible. Dressings may be left on noninfected 2° burns until healing takes place, usually in about 2 weeks. If the surface becomes infected, apply triple antibiotic ointment every 12 hours. Always change the dressing if it becomes wet. Oral antibiotics should be avoided unless an infection develops. Ruptured blisters with sloughed skin should be covered with triple antibiotic ointment. If an infection does occur, use the Sumycin 250 mg, 1 tablet every 6 hours from the Rx kit. Treatment of pain with Percogesic, 2 tablets every 4 to 6 hours from the Rx kit, or Tylenol #3 every 4 to 6 hours from the Rx kit should be adequate.

B. *THIRD DEGREE BURNS (AND DEEP SECOND DEGREE BURNS EXCEPT ON FACE AND HANDS) INVOLVING LESS THAN 15% OF AN ADULT (10% OF CHILD)* -- Generally these patients do not require treatment for shock. Management of the actual burn is as outlined above. A third degree burn of more than 1/2 square inch will require skin grafting. In the meantime dressings will have to be applied and infection prevented or treated as above. The triple antibiotic ointment should be applied from the start.

C. *THIRD DEGREE AND EXTENSIVE SECOND DEGREE BURNS INVOLVING MORE THAN 15% OF AN ADULT (10% OF A CHILD) AND SECOND DEGREE BURNS ON THE FACE OR HANDS -- SHOCK SHOULD BE ANTICIPATED AND TREATMENT BEGUN IMMEDIATELY -- THIS TAKES PRECEDENCE OVER THE WOUND CARE.* Replacement of fluid loss will be the mainstay of shock prevention. The only practical route available to most wilderness travelers will be the oral route. The rule of thumb is to push as much oral fluid as tolerated. Any excess will be urinated off. The amount needed will probably exceed 5 quarts during the first 8-hour period, with another 5 quarts over the next 16 hours. This volume may be adjusted depending upon the urine flow and pulse rate, the two most easily measured parameters of hypovolemic (low fluid level) shock. The ideal urine flow rate should be 50 ml to 100 ml (1⅔ ounce to 3⅓ ounce) per hour. The pulse rate will be elevated due to pain, but it is still a good indicator of hypovolemic conditions and their correction. In adults the rate should be less than 140/min.; in children less than 180/min. If a blood pressure cuff is available -- a normal or high blood pressure should be maintained. The serious difficulty reached with the oral replacement technique is two-fold. The first is vomiting and the second is inability to keep up with fluid losses via the oral route alone if more than 30% of the body surface area is burned

The replacement fluid would ideally consist of Gatorade or a mixture consisting of 1/3 teaspoon of salt and 1/3 teaspoon of baking soda in one quart of flavored, sweetened water. Avoid the use of potassium rich solutions (orange juice, apple juice) as red blood cell destruction will be raising serum potassium to high levels during the first 24 hours.

Generally patients with less than 20% of their body surface area burned can tolerate fluids very well. If they are not vomiting, those with between 20% and 30% of their body surface area involved can be resuscitated by this method without the need for IV fluid replacement, but the patient will have to be treated for shock with the body placed in a recumbent position -- feet elevated. This individual will certainly be marginally shocky. If the victim is vomiting, he will fall way behind in fluid replacement.

During the second day, the oral fluids may consist of Gatorade and sweetened, flavored water (such as Wylers). Watch urine flow to determine the amount of fluids required. On the third day, the patient should be given a moderately high carbohydrate diet, rich in protein. Approximately 200 mg of Vitamin C and substantial Vitamin B complex should be given per day. This would equal about 4 each One-A-Day multiple Vitamin (Miles) or equivalent. Avoid an excessive amount of carbohydrate during the first few days, as a fatal false diabetes may result. Relieve pain with two Percogesic every 4 hours from the nonRx kit or 1 or 2 Tylenol #3 from the Rx kit -- on an as-needed basis. Avoid the use of oral (or injectable antibiotics) to prevent wound infection. If an infection develops, then you may start what you have available, namely from the Rx kit, Sumycin 250 mg, 2 tablets every 6 hours. Treat the burn by leaving it open to the air and applying triple antibiotic ointment. This is not the ideal burn ointment; Silvadene (an Rx item) happens to be my favorite, but it will probably not be available. Occlusive dressings must not be used. The ointment may be placed on thick gauze dressings which are then held against the wound with a single layer of gauze roll dressing. The wound should be cleaned and debrided daily, removing the dead tissue. These patients must obviously be evacuated as soon as possible.

IV fluid replacement would, of course, require sterile needle, IV tubing administration set, and IV fluids. The IV fluid for the first 24 hours should consist solely of Ringer's lactate in an amount calculated by multiplying the patient's weight in kilograms times the total percent of the body surface area burned -- not a maximum of 50% as many formulae have previously recommended. Prior to 24 hours post burn, the capillary leakage of plasma will make use of this substance ineffective -- a tolerable equilibrium will be established. The essential management during that first 24 hours is adequate Ringer's lactate replacement. Since each liter of Ringer's lactate contains 75 ml to 100 ml of free water, it is also not necessary to add D5W during that first day. During the fourth 8 hour period (24 hour to 32 hour post-burn), plasma expansion should be completely provided. The amount of plasma depends upon the extent of the burn.

% burn	Plasma Required for 155 pound man
20 to 40	0 to 500 ml
40 to 60	500 to 1700 ml
60 to 80	1000 to 3000 ml
greater than 80	1500 to 3500 ml

Following the administration of the above, no further volume expansion will normally be required. The daily insensible water losses will have to be replaced. Generally this can revert to the oral (by mouth) replacement method. Due to increased insensible loss through burned skin, this amount should be increased to 3 quarts per day (see further discussion in section on WATER CONSUMPTION, Page 65). It should be obvious from the above, that the wilderness medic, without aid of IV fluids and equipment and without proper sterile environment, has little chance of saving a victim with greater than 30% body burns, that 20% to 30% burn victims have a marginal chance, primarily dependent upon the amount of vomiting, while victims with less than 15% burn, 1° and 2°, should fare well. If limited IV solutions are to be carried, the ideal would be Ringer's lactate in collapsible bags. Plasma comes in glass bottles and costs about $40 per bottle. Refrigeration is not required.

DIABETES MANAGEMENT -- A diabetic child or adult can have an active outdoor life, but learning to control their diabetes is an essential process to be worked out between that individual and his physician. The increased caloric requirement of wilderness exercise may range easily to an extra 2,000 calories per day, yet insulin dosage requirements may drop as much as 50%. Trip partners must be able to identify the signs of hypoglycemia -- staggering gait, slurred speech, clumsy movements -- and know the proper treatment -- i.e. oral carbohydrates or sugar candies and the use of injectable glucagon (if the patient becomes unconscious). Urine of diabetic outdoorsmen must be tested at least twice daily to confirm control of sugar. This testing should preclude a gradual accumulation of too much blood sugar, which can result in unconsciousness in its far advanced stage. This gradual accumulation will cause massive sugar spillage in the urine, and finally the spillage of ketone bodies, providing the patient ample time to correct insulin dosage to prevent hyperglycemic (too much blood sugar) episodes.

Storage of insulin in the wilderness, where it foregoes recommended refrigeration, is not a major problem so long as the supply is fresh and direct sunlight and excessive heat is avoided. Syringes, alcohol prep pads, Keto-diastix urine test strips, insulin and glucagon are light additions to the wilderness medical kit.

DIFFICULTY BREATHING --

If no breathing is present -- from whatever cause --
refer to **ARTIFICIAL RESPIRATION, Page 41.**

If no heart beat is present -- from whatever cause --
refer to **CARDIAC COMPRESSION Page 42.**

If the difficulty starts at high altitude (above 6,500 feet),
refer to the section on **HIGH ALTITUDE ILLNESS, Page 50.**

If the difficulty starts under cold conditions, or conditions of cold weather exposure (under 45° F),
refer to **HYPOTHERMIA, Page 52.**

If body oral temperature is over 100° F and cough is present --
refer to **PNEUMONIA/BRONCHITIS, Page 48.**

If pain is of sudden onset, for no apparent reason, pain in one area made worse with breathing --
refer to **PNEUMOTHORAX, Page 49.**

If associated with pressure feeling, or ache in middle chest, possibly radiating into neck or arm, made worse with exertion and easing with rest; patient sweating, no temp --
refer to **CARDIAC, Page 44.**

ARTIFICIAL RESPIRATION -- The best way to provide artificial respiration is by using the mouth-to-mouth technique. If the victim is not lying flat on his back, roll him over, moving the entire body at one time as a total unit. The victim should be shaken by the shoulder to make sure that he is unconscious. The rescuer should place his face near the victim's to ascertain whether or not air movement is occurring through the mouth or nose. If breathing is absent, the oropharynx and mouth should be cleared of foreign material (snow, mucus, dental plates, vomit, etc.) by inserting the fingers into the mouth and scooping this material out. To open the victim's airway, lift the neck gently with one hand while pushing down on the forehead with the other to tilt the head back (see *Figure 4*). This will place tension on the tongue and throat structures to insure the air passage is open. This opening of the air passage may be all that is required to allow the victim to start breathing again. If opening the airway does not cause spontaneous breathing, start mouth-to-mouth resuscitation. Take the hand which is on the victim's forehead and turn it so that you can pinch the victim's nose shut while still keeping the heel of the hand in place on the forehead to maintain head tilt (see *Figure 5*). The other hand

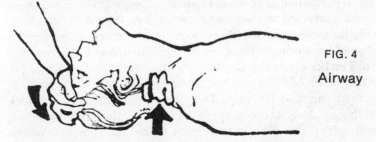

FIG. 4
Airway

Reprinted from the Supplement to Journal of the American Medical Association, Feb. 18, 1974. Copyright 1974, the American Medical Association. Reprinted with permission from the American Heart Association.

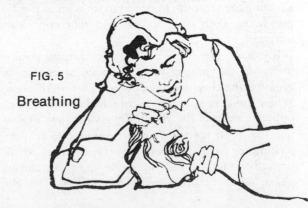

FIG. 5
Breathing

should remain under the victim's neck, lifting up to maintain a patent airway. Immediately give four quick, full breaths in rapid succession using this mouth-to-mouth method. This inflates the victim's lungs and allows for better oxygen transfer. The routine used is for the rescuer to inhale, place his mouth over the victim's open mouth and exhale with enough force to cause the victim's chest to rise -- pinching the nostrils with the hand pushing down on the forehead and lifting under the neck with the other hand. These breaths are repeated every five seconds. In children, don't pinch the nostrils, but place your mouth over both their mouth and nose, giving one small breath every three seconds. If a victim may have a broken neck, avoid pressing down upon the forehead and lifting on the neck, but take the hand that would be lifting under the neck and grasp the lower jaw, pulling it down and open.

CARDIAC COMPRESSION -- Check the victim's carotid pulse. This is easily found by placing your hand on the voice box (larynx). Slide the tips of your fingers into the groove beside the voice box and feel for the pulse -- this is where the carotid artery can easily be palpated. If the pulse cannot be felt, the rescuer must provide artificial circulation in addition to artificial respiration. This is best done with external cardiac compression (see *Figure 6*). Kneel at the victim's side near his chest, locating the notch at the lowest portion of his sternum. Place the heel of one hand on the sternum 1½ to 2 inches above this notch. Place the other hand on top of the one that is in position and the sternum. Be sure to keep your fingers off the ribs. The easiest way to prevent this is to interlock your fingers, thus keeping them confined to the sternum. With your shoulders directly over the victim's sternum, compress downward keeping your arms straight. Depress the sternum 1½ to 2 inches for an average adult victim. Relax the pressure completely, keeping your hands in contact with the sternum at all times, but allowing the sternum to return to its normal position between compressions. Both compression and relaxation should be of equal duration.

If you are providing both artificial respiration and cardiac compression, the proper ratio is 15 chest compressions to 2 quick breaths, the compressions being at a rate of about 80 per minute. When there is another rescuer to help you, position yourself on opposite sides of the victim if possible (see *Figure 7*). The illustration has both rescuers on the same side to better illustrate the technique. The person providing the artificial respiration (mouth-to-mouth) will interpose a breath during the relaxation phase of every 5th chest compression. The chest compression

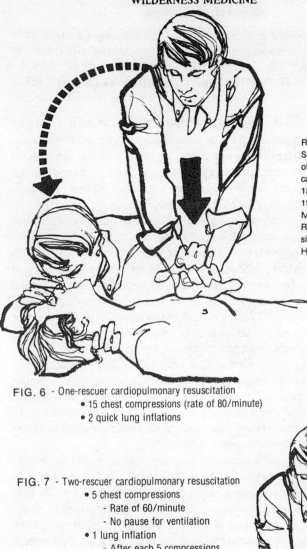

FIG. 6 - One-rescuer cardiopulmonary resuscitation
- 15 chest compressions (rate of 80/minute)
- 2 quick lung inflations

FIG. 7 - Two-rescuer cardiopulmonary resuscitation
- 5 chest compressions
  - Rate of 60/minute
  - No pause for ventilation
- 1 lung inflation
  - After each 5 compressions
  - Interposed between compressions

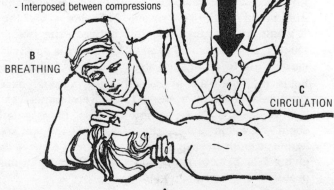

B
BREATHING

C
CIRCULATION

A
AIRWAY

should be performed at a rate of 60 per minute. Being too aggressive with your compression may cause numerous rib fractures. THE ONLY WAY TO LEARN THIS TECHNIQUE IS TO TAKE A CPR COURSE -- IT CANNOT BE PROPERLY SELF-TAUGHT.

CARDIAC -- MYOCARDIAL INFARCTION -- so-called "Heart Attack". The symptoms of chest heaviness or pain with exertion; pain or ache radiating into the neck, generally along the carotid artery or into the arms; sweating; clammy, pale appearance; shortness of breath -- are fairly classic for a cardiac victim. The only thing which can be done for this individual is rest. Position the victim for optimum comfort, generally with his head elevated about 45°. In many cases, even with an electrocardiogram it is impossible for a trained physician to determine whether or not an individual is having a cardiac problem. When in doubt -- rest the patient and try to evacuate without having him do any of the work -- *treat as a total invalid*. If you are carrying the full wilderness Rx medical kit, give him Tylenol #3 for pain and Phenergan 25 mg to prevent nausea and help sedate the victim. If pain is severe, give 2 of the Tylenol #3. The Xylocaine (which you are carrying for local infiltration of lacerations to numb them) is very useful in preventing cardiac arrhythmias (or improper beats). By placing a tourniquet around the arm you may be able to make the veins on the forearm or back of the hand swell. If so, it may be rather easy to inject directly and slowly into one of the veins, a shot containing 5cc of the infiltration Xylocaine (2% plain solution).

This is not the ideal Xylocaine mixture, but it would be better than nothing. In the case of the obvious, sick cardiac patient, do not hesitate to do this. Repeat with another 5cc IV bolus in 20 minutes. The remaining Xylocaine can be given to the patient in doses of 2.5cc each, 3 hours apart. If you are unable to perform the IV puncture, the use of intramuscular Xylocaine may be performed. The normal dose would be 300 mg in the shoulder muscle (deltoid). This would require an awesome 15cc shot or half the entire bottle. It would be best to divide this between the two shoulders. Obviously, a concentrated form of Xylocaine is specially prepared for cardiac use to avoid such large quantities being used IV. The IV bolus would not be a problem with volume, except that your syringe is too small, necessitating several punctures. If some of it infiltrates and does not get into the vein, there is nothing to worry about -- it would cause no tissue damage and you are faced with a heroic attempt to save a life in any event. Repeat the Tylenol #3, giving 1 or 2 every 3 to 4 hours. The Phenergan may also be repeated every 4 hours.

CHOKING -- Even in a fully equipped emergency room, this can be a very difficult, life threatening problem. If the victim is still able to breathe through a partial obstruction and is able to speak or cough effectively, do not interfere with his attempts to expel the foreign body. If the person completely obstructs, is unable to speak, breathe or cough -- perform the following quickly on the conscious victim -- regardless of the victim's position in sitting, standing or lying: 1) 4 back blows; 2) 4 manual thrusts; 3) alternate back blows and manual thrusts until effective or the victim becomes unconscious. If the victim *does* become unconscious, place him on his back, face up. Open the airway and attempt to ventilate. If unsuccessful, roll him onto his side and deliver 4 back blows, 4 manual thrusts. Then probe the mouth with the fingers and again attempt to ventilate. Be persistent. It may be necessary to repeat these steps -- doing so will be the victim's *only* hope of survival at this point. The manual thrusts mentioned are the Heimlich maneuver or variations thereof.

MANUAL THRUST TECHNIQUE -- Ideally, the victim is stood up, grabbed from behind with both arms around his waist and hands interlocked, shoving both fists into the upper abdomen and chest beneath the sternum. A vigorous thrusting squeeze hopefully will cause remaining air in the lungs to expel the foreign body from the clogged airway, much as a cork is shot from an air gun. Any variation of this theme, to thus compress the air suddenly in the chest and force the debris out of the airway, is essential. Dr. Heimlich feels that the back blows may further lodge debris in the airway and that the thrust technique should be applied first. Were these maneuvers to fail and the debris were located above the trachea, a tracheostomy would be life saving. Probably the best field expedient technique is the cricothyrotomy.

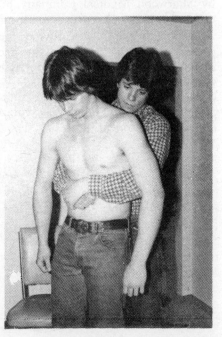

FIG. 8

CRICOTHYROTOMY -- If the patient is in imminent danger of dying from airway obstruction, the obstruction or damage being at a level of the larynx or above, a rapid field technique to provide an artificial airway that is very dangerous, but less so than the even more dangerous tracheostomy, is the cricothyrotomy. In essence, a hole is placed in the thin cricothyroid membrane and a hollow object is placed in this hole to keep an external airway open. This membrane stretches between the Adam's apple (thyroid cartilage) and the prominent ring just below the Adam's apple, called the cricoid cartilage.

With the patient lying on a flat surface, head extended, prepare the area with antiseptic if there is time. Povidine-iodine or alcohol prep pads would work well, Palpate for the cricothyroid membrane's location between the Adam's apple and cricoid cartilage. Make a vertical stab incision through the outer skin and the membrane. This opening will have to be kept from collapsing with the use of a hollow tube (such as a ball point pen casing, if nothing better is available.) [A cannula made especially for this purpose is manufactured by Becton-Dickenson, the Adelson curved cricothyroidotomy cannula, and can be ordered by your physician through a surgical supply house. This cannula would be anchored in place as per the instructions which come with the device. Another type of device is the Emergency Tracheal Catheter made by Sherwood Medical Company of St. Louis MO 63103. This consists of a needle covered with an external 10 gauge catheter. After puncture of the cricothyroid membrane with the needle, the catheter is left in place and the needle withdrawn. In a similar manner, any large bore needle may be used (12 or 14 gauge -- the lower the number, the larger the needle bore.) After placement, the needle would have to be carefully taped into position to prevent dislodgement (see *Figures 9A, 9B, 9C*). Two needles can be placed

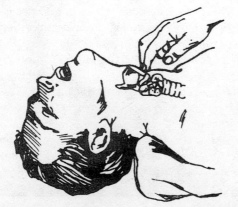

Reprinted by permission from Banyan Emergency Reference Guide, Banyan International Corp., Abilene, Texas.

FIG. 9A

FIG. 9B   FIG. 9C

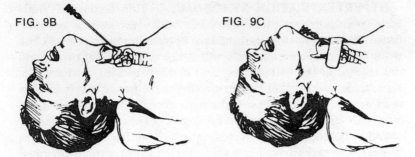

Reprinted by permission from Banyan Emergency Reference Guide, Banyan
International Corp., Abilene, Texas.

side by side to provide better ventilation, especially if oxygen is
not available to enrich the mixture the patient is breathing).

There are many complications that can result from this
procedure -- the esophagus can be punctured, the cricoid cartilage
and first tracheal ring may be cut, the recurrent laryngeal nerve
may be cut, causing damage to the voice, and even the top of the
lung can be punctured. (It is amazing how high in the neck the top
portions of the lungs are located.)

If the patient recovers well enough not to require cricothyrotomy, just remove the needle or cannula and the wound will seal
itself in short order. Butterfly closures should prove adequate to
approximate the wound.

RAPID HEART RATE -- A very rapid rate of 140 to 220 beats per
minute may be encountered suddenly and without warning in very
healthy individuals. This PAT (paroxysmal atrial tachycardia) has
as its first symptom, frequently, a feeling of profound weakness.
The victim generally stops what he is doing and feels better sitting
down. These attacks are self-limited, but they can be aborted by
one of several maneuvers. Holding one's breath and bearing down
very hard may stop this arrhythmia; closing one's eyes and pressing very firmly on the eyeballs may also work; inducing vomiting
with a finger down the throat also works at times. Feel for the
carotid pulse in the neck and gently press on the enlarged portion
of this vessel, one side at a time -- this also can work. Frequently,
however, the victim must just wait for the attack to pass. This
arrhythmia will sometimes come on after a spate of activity. No
medication is generally required.

A rapid heart rate after trauma or other stress may signify im-
pending shock. The underlying cause should be treated. This may
require fluid replacement or pain medication. Temperature eleva-
tions cause an increase in heart rate of 10 beats per minute for
each degree above normal.

HYPERVENTILATION SYNDROME -- This feeling of panic which results in very rapid breathing, with jerky shallow breaths, causes the victim to lose carbon dioxide from the bloodstream. The resulting respiratory alkalosis will cause a numb feeling around the mouth, in the extremities, and if the breathing pattern persists, it can even lead to violent spasms of the hands and feet. This is a form of hysteria, which while more common in women in their 30's, can also appear in teenagers and healthy young adults. It would be helpful for them to rebreathe their air from a stuff sack to increase the carbon dioxide level in their bloodstream. They need to be reassured and told to slow down the breathing. It is fine for them to draw long, deep breaths -- it is the rapid breathing that blows off so much CO_2. If necessary, from the prescription kit give them Phenergan 25 mg, 2 tablets, or from the nonRx kit, Percogesic, 2 tablets. Both drugs are being used here as anti-anxiety drugs. This symptom in a diabetic is very dangerous, but can be prevented by proper diabetic management. High altitude stress can result in temporary hyperventilation (see pages 50 to 52).

HICCUPS -- These can be started by a variety of causes and are generally self-limited. Persistent hiccups can be a medically important symptom requiring professional evaluation and help in control. Several approaches to their control in camp may be tried -- have the victim hold his breath for as long as possible or rebreathe air from a stuff sack -- these maneuvers raise the carbon dioxide level and help stop the hiccup reflex mechanism. Drinking 5 to 6 ounces of ice water fast sometimes works; one may also close his eyes and press firmly on the eyeballs to stimulate the vagal blockage of the hiccup. If these maneuvers do not work, from the Rx kit give the patient Phenergan 25 mg, 2 tablets or, from the nonRx kit give him Percogesic, 2 tablets. Then let him rest and try to avoid bothering him until bedtime. If still symptomatic at that point, have him rebreathe the air from inside his sleeping bag, to raise the carbon dioxide level and muffle the sounds.

PNEUMONIA -- BRONCHITIS -- Infection of the airways into the lung (bronchitis) and its extension into the air sacs of the lung (pneumonia) will cause very high fever, persistent cough, frequently producing phlegm stained with blood, and cause prostration of the victim. Treat the fever with aspirin or Percogesic from the nonRx kit. The severe pain (pleurisy) and cough can be controlled with the Tylenol #3 in the Rx kit. The codeine in the Tylenol #3 is a very effective cough suppressant and is the active ingredient in most of the prescription cough medications. The dosage of these cough preparations generally contains 6 mg of codeine, the

Tylenol #3 has 30 mg per tablet. The fever will require the administration of too much Tylenol to use the Tylenol #3 for this purpose. Give 1 Tylenol #3 with one 5 grain aspirin or Percogesic every 4 hours to fight the fever. Cool with cloth over the forehead as needed. Do not bundle the patient with a very high fever, as this will only drive the temperature even higher. The shivering cold feeling that the patient has is only proof that his thermal control mechanism is out of adjustment -- trust the thermometer or the back of your hand to follow temperature. Encourage the victim to take fluids, as fever and coughing lead to dehydration which will only cause the bronchioles to fill with a tenacious mess. Force fluids to prevent this sputum from plugging up sections of the lung field. Eight glasses of water (64 ounces of fluid total) per day should be adequate.

Provide antibiotic, Sumycin 500 mg, 4 times daily until the fever breaks, then 250 mg, 4 times daily for another 5 to 7 days. Alternatively, use EES 400, 4 times daily. Rest is essential. Prepare a sheltered camp for the victim as best as circumstances permit.

PNEUMOTHORAX -- Even in very healthy young adults and teenagers, it is possible for a bleb on the lung to break -- for no apparent reason -- and fill a portion of the chest cavity with air, thus collapsing part of one lung. A minor pneumothorax will also spontaneously take care of itself, with the air being reabsorbed and the lung re-expanding over 3 to 5 days. The classic sign of decreased breath sounds over the area of the collaspe will be very difficult for the untrained observer, even with a stethoscope. But listen first to one side of the chest and then the other to see if there is a difference. Part of the difficulty lies in the fact that patients with chest pain do not breath deeply and all breath sounds are decreased. Other parts of the physical exam are even more subtle. In unexplained severe chest pain in an otherwise healthy individual, at normal altitude, this might be the cause.

Severe pneumothorax will have to be treated by a physician with removal of the trapped air with a large syringe, flutter valve, or by other methods currently employed in a hospital setting. If pain is severe and breathing difficult, the only choice is evacuation of the victim. From the Rx kit, provide 1 or 2 Tylenol #3 every 4 hours or, from the nonRx kit use Percogesic, 2 tablets every 4 hours.

LIGHTNING -- Lightning bolts cause damage in humans with tissue burns from the heat of the powerful current and by disruption of organ function due to electrical confusion. As the skin has fairly high resistance to electricity, it is at the entrance and exit points from the skin that heat and subsequent burns develop. The current may pass along the low resistance, liquid pathways of the body doing very little damage at all. Wet skin provides less resistance and burns may be minimal -- or the burn can be a third degree char. The disruption to the cardiopulmonary system is the most urgent medical emergency. People screaming from burns, after an electrical bolt has struck, are already out of the immediate danger point -- their wounds may be dressed as indicated under BURNS.

Experiments on animals show that electrical shocks can stop the heart, with a normal rhythm starting spontaneously -- in many instances -- in a short time. The respiratory system, however, may be shut down for 5 to 6 hours before being able to resume its normal rhythm. The most essential point in attending unconscious victims of a lightning strike -- or electrocution in general -- is that after hours of cardiopulmonary resuscitation the victim may suddenly make a recovery -- and make a complete recovery at that. These victims may be physiologically dead, with wide, fixed pupils, lack of respiration and cardiac activity, flaccid muscles -- yet with adequate external cardiac massage and mouth-to-mouth pulmonary resuscitation, total recovery may be achieved. One out of three such victims will still die, but the rescue party shoud not give up until they are physically unable to continue CPR.

HIGH ALTITUDE ILLNESS -- The three major clinical manifestations of this disease complex are outlined below:

ACUTE MOUNTAIN SICKNESS (AMS) - Rarely encountered below 2,000 meters (6,500 feet), it is common in persons going above 3,000 meters (10,000 feet) without taking the time to acclimatize for altitude. Symptoms beginning soon after ascent consist of headache (often severe), nausea, vomiting, shortness of breath, weakness, sleep disturbance and occasionally, periodic breathing.

Prevention, as with all of the high altitude illness problems, is gradual ascent to an altitude above 9,000 feet and light physical activity for the first several days. For persons unable to take adequate time for altitude acclimatization, it may be helpful to take acetazolamide (Diamox) 250 mg every 12 hours prior to ascent and continuing the next 3 to 5 days. Dr. Houston, a leading authority on this problem, made this recommendation in 1976 -- but this theory is still experimental.

Treatment is descent to below 2,000 meters, replacement of fluid loss (particularly important if vomiting has occurred) due to the rapid breathing of air with low relative humidity which is always encountered in cold weather, restriction of salt in-take, a high carbohydrate diet and the administration of oxygen. Of these treatments, the descent in altitude is the most important.

HIGH ALTITUDE PULMONARY EDEMA (HAPE) - This problem is rare below 2,500 meters (8,000 feet), but occurs at higher altitudes in those poorly acclimatized. It is more prone to occur in persons between the ages of 5 and 18 (incidence is apparently less than 0.4% in persons over 21 and as high as 6% in those younger), and in persons who have had this problem before or in those who have been altitude acclimatized and who are returning to high altitude after spending two or more weeks at sea level.

Symptoms develop slowly within 24 to 60 hours of arrival at high altitude with shortness of breath, irritating cough, weakness, rapid heart rate and headache which rapidly progress to intractable cough with bloody sputum, low-grade fever and increasing chest congestion.

Descent to lower altitudes is essential and should not be delayed. Additional treatment is rest in sitting position, oxygen, replacement of fluid loss, rotating tourniquet, probably salt restriction and the use of furosemide (Lasix). Tourniquets should be placed on three limbs at a time, not tight enough to occlude the artery, with one tourniquet being removed every 5 to 10 minutes and repositioned on the free limb.

One regimen suggested for the prevention of HAPE for use in susceptible individuals is the administration of 80 mg of Lasix at the time of arrival in high altitude, and 40 to 80 mg of Lasix every 12 hours for the next 36 to 48 hours. This is a massive dose of a very powerful diuretic and should only be taken under the direct care of a physician. It may further complicate the problem of dehydration, which is a persistent problem at high altitude where daily fluid requirements of 4 to 5 liters are the rule. When pulmonary edema develops, its use may be very beneficial.

Another medication used frequently is morphine sulfate 15 mg by intramuscular injection.

CEREBRAL EDEMA (CE) - This is a less common event than the AMS and HAPE just mentioned, but it is more dangerous. Death has occurred from CE at altitudes as low as 2,500 meters (8,000 feet,) but CE is rare below 3,500 meters (11,500 feet.) The symptoms are increasingly severe headache, mental confusion, emotional behavior, hallucinations, unstable gait, loss of vision, loss of dexterity and facial muscle paralysis. The victim may fall into a restless sleep, followed by a deep coma and death.

Descent is essential, oxygen should be administered and the use of dexamethasone (Decadron) 10 mg intravenously, followed by 4 mg every 6 hours intramuscularly until the symptoms subside. Response is noted usually within 12 to 24 hours and the dosage may be reduced after 2 to 4 days and gradually discontinued over a period of 5 to 7 days. This is a very potent drug and should only be used under the direct supervision of a physician. The most important aspect of therapy for this patient is the immediate descent from the altitude.

As can be noted from the above discussions of AMS, HAPE and CE, the symptoms progress rather insidiously. They are not clear-cut, separate diseases -- they often occur together. The essential therapy for each of them is recognition and descent. This is life saving and more valuable than the administration of oxygen or the sophisticated drugs listed above. To prevent them, it is helpful to "climb high, but camp low" -- i.e., spend nights at the lowest camp elevation feasible.

HYPOTHERMIA -- The essential ingredients in surviving this situation are: being prepared to prevent it, recognizing it if it occurs and knowing how to treat it. On the bottom line, it represents the lowering of the body core temperature -- lower it enough, and death will result! Dampness and wind are the most devastating factors to be considered -- even more so than temperature. It is possible to die of hypothermia in temperatures far above freezing. Most hypothermia deaths occur in the 30° to 50° range.

Proper insulation is the most important aspect of protection. By far the most valuable insulator when wet is wool. Wool loses only 40 to 60% of its insulating ability when wet. Protect the head and hands with wool. Wool shirts have little bulk and can be an invaluable addition to a day pack. Polarguard and Holofill II garments and sleeping bags have also proven to be valuable additions to the wilderness armamentarium. Thinsulate appears very promising. Proper nutrition and avoidance of exhaustion are further factors in preventing hypothermia.

The first response that the body has to a hypothermia condition is vasoconstriction in the skin, thus decreasing the flow of blood to the surface -- which, in effect, lowers surface temperature, but preserves the core temperature. If this heat loss continues, the core temperature will begin to fall below 99°.

HYPOTHERMIA

Body Core Temp.	Symptoms
99 to 96	Shivering intense and uncontrollable Unable to perform complex tasks
95 to 91	Violent shivering persists. Difficulty speaking Sluggish thinking; amnesia starts to appear
90 to 86	Shivering decreases - replaced with muscle rigidity Exposed skin blue or puffy Muscle coordination poor; total amnesia Comprehension dull; generally still able to maintain posture and the appearance of psychological contact
85 to 81	Victim becomes irrational - drifts into stupor Pulse and respiration slow; muscles rigid
80 to 78	Unconsciousness. Reflexes cease. Heartbeat erratic.
Below 78	Pulmonary edema; failure of cardiac and respiratory centers. Death.

Treatment is to prevent any further heat loss and immediately add heat to rewarm the victim. The ideal treatment would be to replace the core heat from the inside out, as subjecting the individual to an outside source of heat would cause the surface blood vessels to open and promote circulation to the surface. The initial effect this would have is to dump a load of very cold blood into the already over-cool core. The temperature of blood in the hands and feet may drop 40 to 50 degrees below that of the body's inner core.

Dr. Lathrop, in his excellent book, *HYPOTHERMIA: KILLER OF THE UNPREPARED,* discusses a central reheating technique being developed by the Mountain Rescue Unit of Oregon, in which they have a portable device to administer warm, moist oxygen to the victim. The next most ideal technique is to immerse the victim in a tub of water at 110°F. Dump them in the tub, clothes and all, without wasting time attempting to remove them. Once the patient relaxes, the clothes may be easily removed.

Lacking ability to do that, the following steps should be taken:

Remove the victim from wind and place him in the best shelter available. Replace wet clothing with dry clothing if possible. Insulate the victim from the ground and add heat. If available, strip the victim and place him in a sleeping bag with a stripped rescuer. A hypothermia victim alone in a well insulated sleeping will simply stay cold. If he is conscious, give him warm drinks and candy or sweetened foods, if available. If no sleeping bag or fire is available, have the party huddle together. Avoid the use of alcohol -- this may act as a vasodilator, thus releasing cold surface blood to the core. The only possible use a judicious amount of alcohol would have is when the extremities have been rewarmed and the victim will not be exposed to cold conditions again.

In summary, prevention is the key to avoiding death from hypothermia. Dr. Lathrop lists six steps to the prevention process. 1) Be aware of how insidious wet, wind and cold can be - avoid unnecessary exposure; 2) Dress for warmth - prepare against wet and wind, remembering wool is your best friend; 3) Have adequate nutrition; 4) Carry emergency bivouac gear, such as a tube or tarp; 5) Bivouac early before coordination and judgment are decreased -- know when to quit the struggle against the elements and prepare a camp; 6) Keep active using isometric contractions of various muscle groups to generate heat until desired warmth is produced.

Anyone going outdoors at any time of the year should read Dr. Lathrop's book (see listing in Bibliography).

FROST NIP - Frost nip, or light frostbite, can be readily treated in the field if recognized early enough. When detected, you should cup your hands and blow upon the affected parts to effect total rewarming. Under identical exposure conditons, some people are more prone to this than others. On one of my trips into subarctic Canada, one of my companions almost constantly frost-nipped his nose at rather mild temperatures (—20°F.) We repeatedly had to warn him, as he seemed oblivious to the fact that the tip of his nose was literally frosted white.

FROSTBITE -- Frostbite represents freezing of skin tissue. Traditionally, several degrees of frostbite are recognized, but the treatment for all is the same and the actual degree of severity will not be known until after the patient has been treated and the amount of damage then (readily) identified.

For victims with deep frostbite, rapid warming is the most effective treatment. Refreezing would result in substantial tissue loss. The frozen part should not be thawed if there is any possibility of refreezing the part. Also, once the victim has been thawed, very careful management of the thawed part is required. The patient actually becomes a stretcher case if the foot is involved. For that reason, it may be necessary to leave the foot or leg(s) frozen and allow the victim to walk back to the evacuation point or facility where the thawing will take place. Peter Freuchen, the great Greenland explorer, once walked days and miles keeping one leg frozen, knowing that when the leg thawed, he would be helpless.

When superficial frostbite is suspected, thaw immediately so that it does not become a more serious, deep frostbite. Warm the hands by withdrawing them into the parka through the sleeves -- avoid opening the front of the parka to minimize heat loss. Feet should be thawed against a companion or cupped in your own hands in a roomy sleeping bag, or otherwise in an insulated environment.

The specific therapy for a deep frozen extremity is rapid thawing in warm water (approx. 110°F.) This thawing may take 20 to 30 minutes, but it should be continued until all paleness of the tips of the fingers or toes has turned to pink or burgundy red, but no longer. This will be very painful and will require pain medication (Rx Tylenol #3, 2 tablets at the start of the procedure)..

Avoid opening the blisters that form. Do not cut skin away, but allow the digits to autoamputate over the next *3 months.* Blisters will usually last 2 to 3 weeks -- these must be treated with care to prevent infections (best done in a hospital with gloved attendants).

A black carapace will form in severe frostbite. This is actually a form of dry gangrene. This carapace will gradually fall off with amazingly good healing beneath -- efforts to hasten the carapace removal generally result in infection, delay in healing and increased loss of tissue. Leave these blackened areas alone. The black carapace separation can take over six months, but it is worth the wait. Without surgical interference, most frostbite wounds heal in six months to a year. All persons heading into the bush should already have had their tetanus booster (within the previous 10 years). Treat for shock routinely with elevation of feet or lowering of head, as this will frequently occur when these people enter a warm environment.

If a frozen member has thawed and the patient must be transported, use cotton between toes (or fluff sterile gauze from the emergency kit and place between toes) and cover other areas with a loose bandage to protect the skin during sleeping bag stretcher evacuation. If fracture also exists, immobilize when in the field, loosely so as not to impair the circulation any further.

FROZEN LUNG -- or pulmonary chilling, more properly, as no tissue is actually frozen, occurs when breathing rapidly at very low temperatures, generally below —20°F. There is burning pain, sometimes coughing of blood, frequently asthmatic wheezing and, with irritation of the diaphragm, pain in the shoulder(s) and upper stomach that may last for 1 to 2 weeks. The treatment is bed rest, steam inhalations, drinking extra water, humidification of quarters and no smoking. Avoid by using parka hoods, face masks or breathing through mufflers which allow the rebreathing of warmed, humidified, expired air.

IMMERSION FOOT - This results from wet, cool conditions with temperature exposures from 68°F (20°C) down to freezing. There are two stages of this problem: the first stage, in which the foot is cold, swollen, waxy, mottled with dark burgundy to blue splotches. This foot is resilient to palpation, whereas the frozen foot is very hard. Skin is sodden and friable. Loss of feeling makes walking difficult. The second stage lasts for days to weeks. The feet are swollen, red and hot; blisters form; infection and gangrene are common.

To prevent this problem, avoid non-breathing (rubber) footwear when possible, dry the feet and change wool socks when feet get wet or sweaty (every 3 to 4 hours, if necessary,) periodically elevate, air, dry, massage the feet to promote circulation. Avoid tight, constricting clothing.

Treatment differs from frostbite and hypothermia in the following ways: 1) Give the patient 10 grains of aspirin every 6 hours to help decrease platelet adhesion and clotting ability of the blood, 2) Give additional Tylenol #3 every 4 hours for pain, but discontinue as soon as possible, 3) Provide an ounce of hard liquor (30 ml) every hour while awake and 2 ounces (60 ml) every 2 hours during sleeping hours -- to vasodilate or increase the flow of blood to the feet. If you are unsure whether or not you are dealing with immersion foot or frostbite, or if you may have suffered both, treat as for frostbite.

CHILBLAINS -- This results from exposure of dry skin to temperatures from low 60°F to freezing. The skin is red, swollen, frequently tender and itching. This is the mildest form of cold injury, no tissue loss results. Treatment is the prevention of further exposure with protective clothing over bare skin and the use of ointments if available, such as A & D Ointment or Vaseline (white petrolatum).

COLD WATER IMMERSION -- Sea water will freeze at 28.6°F (—2°C.) A human immersed in water this cold will have his breath knocked out; after initial shivering, the body goes into a spasm of flexion with hands and knees under the chin and all voluntary control of muscle is lost. The hands are useless in 1 to 5 minutes. Loss of ability to breathe is caused by spasm of trunk muscles. Consciousness lasts from 5 to 7 minutes, with death occuring in 10 to 20 minutes. In waters under 45°F, violent exercise and a frantic attempt to get out of the water is your best chance. Get on land or stable ice immediately and roll in the snow, then get on your feet and keep in aggressive motion until the nearest shelter can be reached. The frozen outer clothing may act as a windbreak; regardless, this aggressive action will be all that will save you. In water over 45°F in conventional clothing, it is best to exert as little activity as possible. Convection loss of heat by moving water is lessened and you will live longer. Protection of the back of the neck and head is vital in both cases. (This is true of hypothermia on dry land as well as exposure to cold water). Recovery of victims is as discussed under HYPOTHERMIA.

HEAT STRESS -- High environmental temperatures are frequently aggravated by the amount of work being done, the humidity, reflection of heat from rock, sand or other structures (even snow!) and the lack of air movement. It takes a human approximately 5 to 7 days to become heat acclimated. Once heat stress adaptation takes place, there will be a decrease in the loss of salt in the sweat produced, thus conserving electrolytes. Another major change that occurs is the rapid formation of sweat and the formation of larger quantities of sweat. Thus, the body is able to start its response to an elevation in the core temperature more rapidly and to utilize its efficient cooling mechanism, sweating, more fully and with less electrolyte disturbance to the body.

Impregnated salt tablets are designed to cause less nausea than straight salt. Specially prepared electrolyte solutions have been manufactured, such as Gatorade, in powder form for reconstitution on the trail, which are palatable and serve the same purpose. Additionally, these solutions contain glucose which aids the rapid uptake of water from the digestive system. Under maximal exertion conditions, it may be necessary to imbibe 3 pints of water per hour and additionally to require 3 to 5 grams of salt per day (this would represent 5 to 7 ten grain salt tablets. Salt tablets currently available are either 5 grain or 10 grain. Be sure to check their strength). Thirst may lag behind requirements, so that oral replacement should be voluntarily done before thirst even becomes noticeable. Water deprivation is dangerous and should be avoided.

Taking this problem in reverse, with no water available, how long could a person expect to survive? The answer is generally dependent upon the temperature and the amount of activity. At a temperature of 120°F with no water available, the victim would expect to survive about 2 days (regardless of activity). This temperature is so high that survival would not be increased beyond 2 days by even 4 quarts of water. Ten quarts might provide an extra day. At 90°F with no water, the person could survive about 5 days if he walked during the day, 7 days if travel was only at night or if no travel was undertaken at all. With 4 quarts of water, survival would extend to 6½ days for day travel and to 10 days for night travel. With 10 quarts, days of survival would increase to 8 and 15 respectively. If the highest temperature was 60°F, with no water, the active person could expect to survive 8 days, the inactive person 10 days.

HEAT CRAMPS -- The excess of sweating caused by a hot environment, especially in a non-heat adapted individual, carries with it the electrolyte sodium chloride. This salt depletion can result in nausea, twitching of muscle groups and at times severe cramping of abdominal muscles, legs, or elsewhere.

Treatment consists of stretching the muscles involved (avoid aggressive massage), resting in a cool environment, and replacing salt losses. Generally 10 to 15 grams of salt and generous water replacement should prevent their returning.

HEAT EXHAUSTION -- This is a classic example of SHOCK, but in this case encountered while working in a hot environment. The body has dilated the blood vessels in the skin, hoping to divert heat from the core to the surface for cooling. However, this dilation is so pronounced, coupled with the profuse sweating and loss of fluid -- also a part of the cooling process, that the blood pressure to the entire system falls too low to adequately supply the brain and the visceral organs. The patient will have a rapid heart rate, and will have the other findings associated with shock: Pale color, nausea, dizziness, headache, and a light-headed feeling. Generally the patient is sweating profusely, but this may not be the case. The temperature is as usual in shock, namely it may be low, normal, or mildly elevated.

Treat as for shock. Have the patient lie down immediately, elevate the feet to increase the blood supply to the head, cover if body temperature is cool or the skin clammy. Also, provide copious water; 10 to 15 grams of salt would also be helpful, but water is the most important, minimum of 1 to 2 quarts. Obviously, fluids can only be administered if the patient is conscious. If unconscious, elevate the feet 3 feet above head level, protect from aspiration of vomit, try to revive with an ammonia inhalant. Then give water when the sensorium clears (patient awakens).

HEAT STROKE (SUN STROKE) -- This represents the complete breakdown of the heat control process (thermal regulation) in the human body. There is a total loss of the ability to sweat, core temperatures rise over 105°F *rapidly* and will soon exceed 115°F and result in death if this is not treated aggressively. THIS IS A TRUE EMERGENCY. The patient will be confused and rapidly become unconscious. Immediately move into shade or erect a hasty barrier for shade. The U.S. Steel Mill employs immediate immersion in ice water to lower the temperature. Once the core temperature lowers to 102°F the victim is removed and the temperature carefully monitored. It may continue to fall or suddenly raise again.

Further cooling with wet cloths may suffice. IV solutions of normal saline are started in the clinic setting -- in the wilderness, douse the victim with the coolest water possible. Massage limbs to allow the cooler blood of the extremities to return to core circulation more readily.

Due to the extreme emergency of this situation (which is related in severity to cardiac and pulmonary standstill) it is better to risk cold injury than to fry the patient's brain. Sacrifice your water supply -- if necessary, urinate on the victim, fan and massage to provide the best coolant effect possible. This person should be evacuated as soon as possible, for his thermal regulation mechanism is quite literally unstable and will be labial for an undeterminable length of time. He should be placed under a physician's care as soon as possible. Terminate the expedition, if necessary, to evacuate.

PRICKLY HEAT -- This is a heat rash caused by the entrapment of sweat in glands in the skin. This can result in irritation and frequently severe itching. Treatment includes cooling and drying the involved area and avoiding conditions that may induce sweating for awhile. Topical medications are less effective than the steps just mentioned, but a good topical would be any of the corticosteroid lotions or creams (an example would be cordran lotion or cream). This cream could be applied three times a day during the symptomatic period. From the Rx kit, apply a light coat of the Cortisporin ointment every 8 hours.

SEVERE STOMACH PAIN — ACUTE ABDOMEN — APPENDICITIS --

An acute abdomen is the term applied to a medical/surgical emergency requiring rapid surgical intervention for the patient's survival. Included in this category are such disasters as appendicitis and perforated ulcer.

Generally wilderness travelers have a phobia about appendicitis; this is the problem I am most frequently asked about in discussions of the subject. The classic presentation of this illness is the vague feeling of discomfort around the umbilicus (navel). Temperature may be low grade, 99.6 to 100.6, at first. Within a matter of hours the discomfort turns to pain and localizes in the right lower quadrant, most frequently on a point 1/3 of the way between the navel and the very top of the right pelvic bone (anterior-superior iliac spine). This pain syndrome can be elicited from the patient by asking two questions: When did you first start hurting, and where did you hurt? (belly button); Now where do you hurt? (right lower quadrant as described). Those answers mean appendicitis until it is ruled out.

Sometimes even full laboratory and x-ray facilities can do no better in evaluating this diagnosis -- the ultimate answer will come from surgical exploration. Now if a surgeon has doubts, he might wait, with the patient safely in a hospital or at home under close supervision. But the patient with those symptoms should certainly be taken to a surgeon as soon as possible.

In the examination of the acute abdomen, several maneuvers can assess the seriousness of the situation. The first is the determination of guarding to palpation. If the patient has a rigid stomach to gentle pushing, this can mean that extreme tenderness and irritation of the peritoneum, or abdomen wall lining, exists -- use only gentle pushing. If there is an area of the abdomen where it does not hurt to push, apply pressure rather deeply. Suddenly take your hand away -- if pain flares over the area of suspect tenderness, this is called "referred rebound tenderness" and it means that the irritation has reached an advanced stage. This person should be evacuated to surgical help at once.

Now what can you do if you are in the deep bush, say the Back River of Canada, without the faintest hope of evacuating the patient? Move the patient as little as possible. No further prodding of the abdomen should be done, as his only hope is that the appendix will form an abscess that will be walled-off by the bodily defense mechanisms. Give him no food -- provide small amounts of water, Gatorade, fruit drinks as tolerated. With advanced disease the intestines will stop working and the patient will vomit any excess. This will obviously cause a disturbance to the gut and possibly rupture the appendix or the abscess -- however, there is not much that you can do about it.

Dehydration is also a very serious problem and the patient will have to have liquids to survive the ordeal ahead of him. Provide antibiotic from the Rx kit (Sumycin 250 mg tablets, 2 every 4 hours). For pain and fever give Tylenol #3, 2 tablets every 4 hours. To help prevent vomiting and to make the Tylenol #3 work better, also give Phenergan 25 mg every 4 hours. These can be administered with the small amounts of fluid mentioned above.

The abscess should form 24 to 72 hours following onset of the illness. Many surgeons would elect to open and drain this abscess as soon as the patient is brought to their control. Other surgeons would feel that it is best to leave the patient alone at this time and allow the abscess to continue the walling-off process. These surgeons feel that there is so much inflammation present, surgery only complicates the situation further. Within 2 to 3 weeks the patient may be able to move with minimal discomfort. What are the chances of recovery under these conditions? I can find nothing in print. With IV antibiotics and hydration, the survival should be about 80%. It may actually be that high without IV use.

One form of therapy never to be employed when there is a suspicion of appendicitis is the use of a laxative. The action of the laxative may cause disruption of the appendix abscess with resultant generalized peritonitis (massive abdominal infection).

It is currently thought that there is no justification for the prophylactic removal of an appendix in an individual, unless he is planning to move to a very remote area without medical help for an extended period of time and it is known from x-ray that he has a fecolith in the region of the appendix. Otherwise, the possible latter complications of surgical adhesions may well outweigh the "benefit" of such a procedure.

HEART BURN -- Gastritis, the burning sensation, most frequently accompanied by tenderness to palpation just beneath the breast bone or sternum (in the mid-epigastrium) should be aggressively treated at its onset. This irritation can lead to gastric or duodenal ulcer formation. The pain may represent reflux of stomach contents up the esophagus (esophagitis or hiatal hernia) -- this too needs rapid treatment to prevent unnecessary discomfort and possible complications.

The best line of defense is antacid. For wilderness use I recommend carrying tablets of Camalox. They are very powerful for their size (two tablets neutralize 36 mEq of acid). They contain magnesium hydroxide, aluminum hydroxide and calcium carbonate. For routine home use I would avoid constant use of calcium carbonate, but for the wilderness this formulation approach is ideal. Further, the manufacturer has had the foresight to seal these tablets in heavy aluminum foil. Nausea of severe heart burn or ulcer attacks can be helped with Phenergan 25 mg from the Rx kit, 1 tablet every 6 hours, or meclizine 25 mg from the nonRx kit, 1 every 8 hours. Eat multiple meals a day -- frequent munching on pilot biscuits or other bread items may be helpful. If powdered milk is available, use it. A very palatable preparation is "Milkman," produced by Foremost Dairies in California and available from the publisher of this book. The use of anticholinergics, which prevent stomach emptying (such as probanthine), is now being discouraged by some experts, but a specific drug to block acid formation, Tagamet 300 mg, has been released for use in the U.S. Although marketed here only for duodenal ulcer therapy, I have found it very helpful for gastric ulcer and reflux esophagitis (hiatal hernia) treatment as well. If the woodsman frequently experiences ulcer problems, discuss with your physician the possible inclusion in your Wilderness Medical Kit of this Rx item.

HERNIA -- The most common hernia in a male is the inguinal hernia, which is an outpouching of the intestines through a weak area in the abdominal wall located above the penis. This hernia will be produced while straining, either lifting, coughing, sneezing, etc. There will be a sharp pain at the location of the hernia. The patient will note a bulge in the area. This bulge may disappear when he lies on his back and relaxes (i.e. the hernia has reduced). If the intestine in the hernia is squeezed by the abdominal wall to the point that the blood supply is cut off, the hernia is termed a "strangulated" hernia. This is a medical emergency, as the loop of gut in the hernia will die, turn gangrenous, and lead to a generalized peritonitis or abdomen infection -- as discussed under APPENDICITIS. This condition is much worse than an appendicitis and death will result if not treat surgically.

The hernia that fails to reduce, or disappear when the victim relaxes in a recumbant position, is termed "incarcerated". While this may turn into an emergency, it is not one at that point. Most hernia caused by straining in adults will not strangulate. Further straining should be avoided. If lifting items is *necessary*, or while coughing, etc., the victim should protect himself from further tissue damage by pressing against the area with one hand -- thus holding the hernia in reduction. It would be a rather awkward way to carry a canoe.

MOTION SICKNESS -- To prevent and treat motion sickness, a very useful nonRx drug is meclizine 25 mg, taken one hour prior to departure for all day protection. This particular drug is a prescription-only medication when written to cure vertigo associated with inner ear dysfunction (its major brand name for that purpose is Antivert and the prescription generally calls for 12.5 mg or 25 mg 3 times a day) or, from the Rx medical kit use the Phenergan 25 mg, 1 tablet every 6 to 8 hours.

VOMITING -- Nausea and vomiting can be caused by a variety of upsets. Generally, the treatment of vomiting includes the use of an anti-emetic or anti-nausea medication. These are available as rectal suppositories, injections and as pills. Obviously, severe vomiting will make the use of pills rather difficult, but this is still the easiest way to approach the subject for wilderness travel. The rectal suppositories melt very easily and the fewer injectable medications required, the better. Their use is always more risky than the use of oral medications and injectables are subject to freezing, breakage and the necessity for syringe needles, etc. From the Rx kit, use Phenergan 25 mg, 1 tablet every 6 hours. Allow the patient to moisten his lips. Only small amounts of fluid should be allowed at frequent intervals. Avoid solid food until the nausea is under control. The use of Gatorade or a flavored fruit drink is fine or, from the nonRx kit, use meclizine 25 mg, 1 tablet every 9 hours. This is a more frequent interval than the OTC instructions permit, as noted in the section on the Nonprescription (nonRx) Wilderness Medical Kit.

Frequently vomiting may be caused by a severe infection, such as tonsilitis, sinusitis, etc. Correction of the underlying disorder in these cases is the best approach to the therapy of the vomiting and nausea. The nausea induced by high altitude is discussed under HIGH ALTITUDE SICKNESS. Nausea is a frequent complaint of many viral illnesses.

One of particular importance to wilderness travelers in under-developed countries is HEPATITIS caused by the Hepatitis A virus (formerly called infectious hepatitis.) This disease is common and worldwide. Its symptoms vary from a minor flu-like illness to fatal liver failure. It takes two to six weeks to develop the disease from time of contact. After 3 to 10 days of nausea, vomiting, lethargy and fever, the urine will turn dark, followed by a yellow color in the whites of the eyes and in severe cases, yellow skin. This jaundice reaches a peak in 1 to 2 weeks and gradually esolves during a 2 to 4 week recovery phase. Urine, blood and stool should be considered very contaminated -- these must be carefully disposed of to prevent spread of the disease. Personal hygiene helps prevent this spread, but isolation of the patient is not strictly required. In most cases no specific treatment is required -- after a few days appetite generally returns and bed confinement is no longer required. Restrictions of diet have no value.

The patient may safely return to full activity before the jaundice completely resolves -- the best guideline is the disappearance of the lethargy and feeling of illness that appeared in the first stages of the disease. If profound prostration occurs, and certainly when feasible, the trip should be terminated for the patient and he should be placed under medical care. If possible, contacts should receive Gamma-globulin 0.02 ml/kg IM. The use of Gamma-globulin prophylactically is discussed under IMMUNIZATION.

FOOD POISONING -- Eating tainted food can be the cause of violent vomiting and diarrhea. Generally, the vomiting and diarrhea will tend to eliminate the cause of the problem. In fact, stopping these discomforts can lead to further problems by allowing the toxic substances to remain longer within the patient. After the stomach and intestines have obviously been emptied by their unpleasant reactions, it would be appropriate to replace fluid losses and treat diarrhea as described on Pages 68 through 70 and the vomiting as outlined on Page 63.

Prevention is effected by staying alert. Water sources must be known pure or treated as indicated on Pages 66 and 67. Tainted food should be avoided. Once dehydrated or freeze-dried food has been reconstituted, it should be stored as carefully as any fresh, unprocessed food. Be wary of fresh fruits and vegetables in developing countries. Peel all such items, or thoroughly rinse with purified water, or boil for 10 minutes minimum. Often, in countries lacking refrigeration, fruits and vegetables are "freshened" on the way to market by sprinkling these items frequently with water from road side drainage ditches. The use of human fertilizer makes this water very contaminated. This contamination is not eliminated by drying or wiping with a cloth. Certain animal products are tainted in various parts of the world, particularly at specific times of the year. Know the flora and fauna which your expedition plans to utilize from local sources!

TRICHINOSIS is caused by eating improperly cooked meat infected with the cysts of this parasite. It is most common in pigs, bears (particularly Polar Bears) and some marine mammals. Nausea and diarrhea or intestinal cramping may appear within 1 to 2 days, but it generally takes 7 days after ingestion. Swelling of the eyelids is very characteristic on the 11th day. Afterwards, muscle soreness, fever, pain in the eyes and subconjunctival hemmorhage (see Page 27) develop. If enough contaminated food is ingested this can be a fatal disease. Most symptoms disappear in 3 months. Treatment is with pain medication (Percogesic from the nonRx kit or Tylenol #3 from the Rx kit). The use of steroids such as prednisone (6o mg/day for 3 or 4 days, followed by reduced dosage over the next 10 days) is indicated in severe cases. Thiabendazole is a specific drug for use in this condition, given orally in doses of 25 mg/kg of body weight twice daily for 5 to 10 days. The best prevention is cooking suspected meat at 150°F for 30 minutes for each pound of meat.

MENSTRUAL PROBLEMS -- Menstrual flow is best contained with a vaginally inserted pad, but be sure to have had experience with the product chosen prior to heading backcountry with a supply. Most come with waxed disposable paper bags, but an inner bag of plastic should be carried if it will be necessary to pack out discarded pads. Menstrual cramping can generally be controlled with Percogesic, 1 or 2 tablets every 4 to 6 hours from the nonRx kit. From the Rx kit, if necessary, one could use Tylenol #3, 1 tablet every 4 to 6 hours. A prescription product that I have had considerable success in prescribing for this condition is Nalfon, 600 mg. 1 tablet every 6 hours as required. This product is not approved by the FDA for that purpose, as it is designed as an anti-arthritic, but its anti-prostoglandin activities seem to make it a theoretical, as well as practical, pharmacologic agent with great promise in this area. A good nonRx item is Sunril, 1 capsule every 6 hours, maximum use is 10 days in a one month period.

Menorrhagia, either excessive flow or long period of flowage, should be evaluated by a physician to determine if there is an underlying pathology that could or should be corrected. If the problem is simply one of hormone imbalance, this can frequently be corrected with the use of birth control pills with higher amounts of estrogen and lower progestogen content. Again, the physician should be consulted well in advance of the wilderness outing, so that these symptoms will have been brought under control by the time of the expedition.

WATER CONSUMPTION -- The food which we eat on a daily basis contains about 1,000 ml (1.1 quarts) of water. We generally imbibe another 1,200 ml of liquid and we form about 300 ml of water in our body by the oxidation of foods during metabolism. Our losses of water include 800 to 1,000 ml in the urine, 100 ml in stool, and 600 to 1,000 ml as an insensible loss through our lungs and skin. This latter loss does not include sweating. During high environmental temperatures, we may lose 2,000 to 5,000 ml of water beyond urinary losses. This loss must be matched with intake. Persons should not be starved for water -- in fact, drinking should keep ahead of thirst to prevent inadvertent dehydration under heat stress conditions.

When persons have become acclimated to heat stress, they develop a more ready sweating ability and increased sweating rate and an increase in thermal conductivity. For this system to work, adequate supplies of water must be available. With low environmental temperatures our insensible water losses increase due to the difference in relative humidity of the air we breathe. In fact, in arctic travel conditions, a cold glass of water is one of the greatest treats there is!

WATER PURIFICATION -- Amongst the products commercially available for purification of water, there are several mechanical methods -- some new and others ancient -- that are currently in vogue. One of the proven pharmaceuticals used for water purification is Halazone. Regardless of what the 1975 Western Journal of Medicine article on water purification says, these tablets are actually quite stable -- with a shelf life of at least 5 years, even when exposed to temperatures over 100°F occasionally. They turn yellow and have an objectionable odor when they decompose.

Halazone tablets are highly effective virucidal agents and eradicate most common pathogenic bacteria: namely Halazone is effective against E. coli, typhoid, paratyphoid A and B, cholera and shigella. In general, it is less effective against the spores of certain pathogenic protozoans. High organic particulate matter (turbid water source) decreases the tablet's effectiveness, as does alkaline water. It works best in a soft water or slightly acid water Another popular product is Tetraglycine hydroperiodide (trade name of Potable Aqua). This product releases titratable iodine, which is very effective against even protozoan cysts -- in all cases adequate holding time to allow purification is essential. Obtain the cleanest appearing water possible -- increase the holding time if the water is turbid or very cold. Several manufacturers are selling portable filtration devices to help eliminate organic material and to absorb the taste of the iodine or chlorine after water treatment.

In May of 1975 an article in The Western Journal of Medicine advocated the use of a supersaturated water solution of iodine to purify water. In the technique described, a 1 ounce amber bottle was filled with 4 to 8 grams of Iodine, USP grade, and the bottle was then filled with water. This was carried with the camper, who, when needing to use it, would decant off half the water into a 1 liter canteen. The "bottle generator" was refilled for future use, the canteen was left to sit 20 to 30 minutes and the water then consumed. The system has the advantage of lasting a very long time -- the iodine crystals would replenish the saturated solution of water numerous times. It is a highly effective method of killing virus, bacteria and protozoan contaminant. It works better, as all techniques do, with less organic matter in the water and when the water is warm as opposed to near freezing. After the water has set the required time, *and not before,* fruit drink crystals can be added to disguise the taste, or coffee or tea may be prepared from it.

And let's not forget that most primitive friend of ours - fire. Boiling water is one of the safest and least technically difficult methods of preparing water, Dr. Harold Wolf, Head of the Environmental Engineering Program, Civil Engineering Department, Texas A&M University, feels that simply bringing water to a boil, regardless of altitude, ensures the safety of that water to drink. This technique would allow considerable fuel and time saving in the preparation of potable (drinkable) water. It is also possible to boil water under most survival conditions.

Water may be obtained by squeezing any fresh water fish and from some plants. Never drink urine or sea water, as the high solute content of these liquids will only dehydrate you more and make the problem worse. A solar still can be prepared for reprocessing urine, water from grass, etc. -- as indicated in *Figure 10.* In water poor areas, catching rain water may be an essential part of the routine survival. Be careful of melting ice: treat all ice melt water with Halazone Potable Aqua or the iodine crystals as indicated above. There is a very strong chance of contamination of ice deposits.

SOLAR STILL

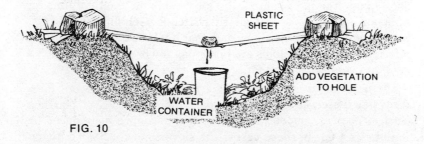

FIG. 10

CONDENSING DRINKABLE WATER FROM VEGETATION
OR CONTAMINATED SOURCES.

HUMAN WASTE DISPOSAL -- This is not only a matter of esthetics, but of primary preventative medicine. Improper waste disposal on the wagon trains heading west in the 1840-1850's caused vast epidemics of cholera in the trains that followed. Unbelievable numbers of people were killed. Even in our wilderness areas, it is widely acknowledged that the cleanest appearing streams are suspect of human contamination. Isle Royal streams are totally polluted with giardia (a human pathogen -- actually a protozoan causing severe diarrhea and illness). Most official campsites in the national park system have toilets constructed. These should *always* be used. Otherwise, human defecation should be buried at least 40 yards from a lakeshore or stream run-off. Use biodegradeable toilet paper, such as one would buy from a camping specialty store or for use in septic tanks. An inexpensive lightweight plastic trowel, ideal for digging a "cat hole," can be purchased at most specialty shops. Some woodsmen prefer to avoid the use of toilet paper and rely upon local moss, plants, etc. to wipe. This is fine if the user isn't wiping with an endangered species or poison ivy! Also, it is very necessary to have adequate water and soap for thorough hand washing. Frankly, I believe it is safer for the ecology and the party to use toilet paper as described. For an expanded discussion of this topic, see Calvin Rutstrum's *CHIPS FROM A WILDERNESS LOG*, Pages 73-76.

DIARRHEA -- Diarrhea is the expulsion of watery stool. This malady can be either a nuisance or an actual threat to life, depending upon its cause and extent. The diarrhea may result from having been constipated too long, in which case the etiology should be readily apparent. This diarrhea is generally of short duration, less than 24 hours. Viral enteritis will also be explosive, but generally short lived. Again, 24 hours is the most common length of time for affliction -- at times, a viral enteritis extends itself for several days, but by then you become suspicious that it might be a more serious infection, unless the stools are becoming fewer (say, only 3 to 5 a day) and somewhat formed.

There are some very powerful drugs available to curtail diarrhea, but these should not be used in certain types of diarrhea (such as cholera, amoebic dysentary, giardiasis, colitis induced by antibiotics.) For in these cases, the slowing of the infected stool passage through the intestines will allow the infectious agent to work its way through the intestines and cause severe complications, such as liver abscesses, etc.

As mentioned, the less serious viral diarrhea is self-limited. If the diarrhea lasts longer than one day, if the fever is high (above

100°F), or if blood is in the stool, become suspicious that a more serious illness has been acquired. Very useful in curtailing cholera, amoebic and bacillary infections is the use of the Sumycin from the Rx kit -- 250 mg 4 times a day. This may safely be started immediately. Recently, it has been proposed that all travelers heading into cholera and other areas famous for "Montezuma's Revenge," should take another tetracycline called Doxycycline (100 mg capsule, 1 daily). This is a very expensive drug, each capsule costing about $1.20. But for expeditions to areas of this nature, well worth carrying it specifically. Otherwise, the Sumycin should be an adequate answer to this problem.

If traveling to Isle Royale or other areas in which *Giardia lamblia* is present, the specific drug of choice to kill this parasite is Flagyl (metronidazole) 250 mg 3 times a day for a week. This drug frequently causes a nauseated feeling. This is the drug which is generally used to combat trichomoniasis vaginal infections in women. It is also useful against amoebic dysentery.

A very safe nonRx drug which may be started immediately without fear of the complications mentioned above is Bacid capsules. These capsules consist of the freeze-dried bacteria called *Lactobacillus acidophilus*. These bacteria can "reseed" the gut and effectively compete with the minor pathogens to curtail diarrhea. I have used this drug many times and have become very satisfied with it. The major drawback is that the manufacturer recommends that the capsules be refrigerated, an impossible nuisance on a wilderness trip. This refrigeration certainly prolongs the storage life of the medication, but as long as the capsules are not exposed to sun, excessive heat or moisture, they will fare very well, even on a wilderness trip of several months. Take 2 capsules every 6 to 12 hours.

The most powerful drug available in the Rx kit is Tylenol #3 containing codeine, to be taken one tablet every 4 to 6 hours to control the cramping and diarrhea. However, this should be used with caution, as previously noted. A popular prescription drug that is specific for diarrhea is Lomotil (taken 2 tablets every 6 hours.) Profound diarrheas from *any* source may cause severe dehydration and electrolyte imbalance. The non-vomiting patient must receive adequate fluid replacement, equaling his stool loss plus about 2 liters per day. The Center for Disease Control has recommended the following oral replacement cocktails to replace the losses of profound diarrhea:

Prepare two separate glasses of the following:

Glass 1) Orange, apple or other fruit juice
(rich in potassium)....................... 8 ounces
Honey or corn syrup (glucose necessary
for absorption of essential salts) .... ½ teaspoon
Salt, table (rich in sodium and chloride) .... 1 pinch

Glass 2) Water (carbonated or boiled) .... 8 ounces
Soda, baking (sodium bicarbonate) .... ¼ teaspoon

Drink alternately from each glass. Supplement with carbonated beverages or water and tea made with boiled or carbonated water as desired. Avoid solid foods and milk until recovery.

It should be noted that the use of Gatorade, available in a powdered form from many backpacking specialty shops, may be used to replace Glass 1, except that the water used must be boiled or carbonated, as mentioned under Glass 2.

In summary, for the general wilderness expedition when diarrhea is encountered and no medical facilities are available, if the temp is low grade and there is no blood in the stool, from the nonRx kit use Bacid capsules, two each four times a day; replace fluid loss with Gatorade and other liquid or, from the prescription kit, use Tylenol #3, 1 tablet every 6 hours. If high temp and/or blood stools are present, treat with Sumycin 500 mg, 4 times a day and use the Bacid capsules. If vomiting is a complication, which it can be under these conditions, give Phenergan 25 mg every 6 hours as necessary (from the Rx kit) or meclizine 25 mg every 8 hours (from the nonRx kit).

TYPHOID FEVER -- This disease is characterized by headache, chills, loss of appetite, backache, constipation, nosebleed and tenderness of the abdomen to palpation. The temperature rises daily for 7 to 10 days. The fever is maintained at a high level for 7 to 10 more days, then drops over the next 10 days. The pulse rate is low for the amount of fever (generally, the pulse rate will increase 10 beats per minute for every 1° of temperature elevation over normal for that individual). With typhoid fever, a pulse rate of 84 may occur with a temperature of 104°F. Between the 7th and 10th day of illness, rose-colored splotches -- which blanche when pressure is applied -- appear in 10% of patients.

The drug of choice for this illness is chloramphenicol, which is a very treacherous drug to use. If an expedition is heading to Mexico or Southeast Asia, it would be best to avoid dependence upon chloramphenicol, as a number of resistant strains have been isolated in these areas. IV Ampicillin (6 grams per day) is the drug of choice in these areas, but an oral medication useful as a back-up drug for penicillin sensitive individuals is Septra (another brand name is Bactrim), 2 tablets 3 times a day. There are very few side effects from this drug. Diarrhea may become important in the latter stages of this illness. Replacement of fluids is especially important during the phases of high fever. Patients with relapses should be given another 5-day course of the Septra. Immunization prior to departure to endemic areas is useful in curtailing the severity of this infection (see pages 104 - 105).

CONSTIPATION -- One of the currently popular wilderness medical texts has instructions on how to break up a fecal impaction digitally (i.e., using your finger to break up a hard stool stuck in the rectum). Don't let it get that far. In healthy young adults (especially teenagers), there may be a reluctance to defecate in the wilderness due to the unusual surroundings, lack of a toilet and perhaps swarms of insects or freezing cold. It is the group leader's responsibility to *make sure* that a trip member does not fecal hoard -- i.e., fail to defecate in a reasonable length of time. Certainly one should be concerned after 3 days of no bowel movements.

To prevent this problem, I always include a stewed fruit at breakfast. The use of hot and cold in the morning will frequently wake up the "gastric-colic reflex" and get things moving perfectly well. If the 5-day mark is approaching, especially if the patient -- and they *have* become a patient at about this point -- is obviously uncomfortable, it may become necessary to use a laxative. From the medical kit (nonRx item) give 1 bisacodyl laxative tablet 5 mg at bedtime. If that fails, the next morning take 2 of the tablets. Under winter conditions, when getting up in sub-zero weather might prove abominable, or under heavy insect conditions, take these tablets in the morning, rather than at night, to preclude this massive inconvenience. Any laxative will cause abdominal cramping, depending upon how strong it is. Be expecting this.

HEMORRHOIDS (PILES) -- These are a type of varicose vein around the rectum. External hemorrhoids are small, rounded purplish masses which enlarge when straining at stool. Unless a clot forms in them, they are soft and nontender. When clots form, they can become very painful, actually excruciating. Hemorrhoids are the most common cause of rectal bleeding, with the blood also appearing on the toilet tissue. The condition can be very painful for about 5 days, after which the clot starts to absorb, the pain decreases and the mass regresses, leaving only small skin tags. Provide the patient with pain medication (nonRx Percogesic, 2 tablets every 4 hours or, Rx Tylenol #3, 1 or 2 tablets every 4 hours). The application of heat is helpful during the acute phase. Heat a cloth in water and apply for 15 minutes 4 times a day if possible. Avoid constipation, as mentioned in that section.

BLADDER INFECTION -- The hallmarks of bladder infection are the urge to urinate frequently, burning upon urination, small amounts of urine being voided with each passage, discomfort in the suprapubic region, the lowest area of the abdomen. Frequently the victim has fever with its attendant chills and muscle ache. In fact, people can become quite ill with a generalized infection caused by numerous bacteria entering their blood stream. At times the urine becomes cloudy and even bloody. Cloudy urine without the above symptoms does NOT mean an infection is present and is frequently normal. The infection can extend to the kidney, at which time the patient also has considerable flank pain, centered at the bottom edge of the ribs along the lateral aspect of the back on the involved side (often both sides). Bladder infections are more common in women than men, they are not an uncommon problem in either sex. One suffering from recurrent infections should be thoroughly evaluated by his physician.

There have been many drugs developed for treating infections of the genito-urinary system. The drug included in the wilderness medical kit is very effective, both for the simple bladder infection, as well as the more severe kidney involvements. Take Sumycin 250 mg, 1 tablet every 6 hours. This medication should be continued for 10 days to make sure that the organism has been eradicated. Symptoms should disappear within 24 to 36 hours, or it may mean that the bacteria is resistant to the antibiotic and another one should be chosen. The back-up drug in the wilderness kit (Erythromycin or EES 400) is not an effective drug for this type of problem. Probably the next most valuable drug for general use would be a broad spectrum penicillin, such as amoxicillin or carbenicillin.

Additional treatment should also consist of drinking copious amounts of fluid, at least *8 quarts per day!* At times, this simple rinsing action may even cure a simple cystitis, but I wouldn't want to count on it if an antibiotic were available. Discomfort may be relieved by Percogesic or, from the Rx kit, a Tylenol #3, but these are seldom required due to the rapid onset of relief following administration of the antibiotic. Percogesic or aspirin will be needed for the fever which accompanies such problems prior to the start of the antibiotic and during the early stages of therapy.

EPIDIDYMITIS AND ORCHITIS -- In males the testicles may become infected (orchitis) or the sperm collecting apparatus forming a cap just above the testicle may become infected (epididymitis). The latter is more common than the former. The hallmark of these problems is pain and swelling of the area.

The patient should be allowed to rest and immediately started on the Sumycin. Use two 250 mg tablets every 6 hours until the symptoms abate, but continue therapy with one 250 mg tablet every 4 hours for at least a total of 10 days. Pain pills will be required for several days. If no response is apparent, the patient may be suffering from a bacteria that is resistant to the antibiotic, or the problem may not be an infection at all. It is possible for the testicle to become twisted, due to a slight congenital defect, with severe pain resulting. This "torsion testicle," as it is called, requires an immediate surgical cure. In the bush this is impossible. Realize that you have a very sick person who will require evacuation and removal of the involved testicle. In the meantime, give the antibiotic, the strongest pain medication available and anti-nausea medication if required. If there is a history of straining prior to onset of the pain, strongly suspect a hernia (see HERNIA.) If the Sumycin is the only antibiotic you are carrying, continue to give it, for several weeks if necessary, until symptoms abate or evacuation is effected.

VENEREAL DISEASE -- The most common of the venereal diseases are gonorrhea and syphilis. The former is easy to diagnose generally in the male, as there is a discharge of greenish yellow pus that increases in intensity. The incubation period, or time for the symptoms to develop from the time of sexual contact, is 2 to 8 days. This disease is transmitted by sexual contact. Women will generally remain asymptomatic (have no symptoms or physical findings to indicate that they are infected).

The drug regimen of choice with this disease is 1 gram of probenecid orally and simultaneously 4.8 million units of Procaine Penicillin by injection. As the latter must be kept refrigerated, it is not suitable for expedition use. The major antibiotic of the Rx kit, Sumycin, is an alternate drug for treating this disease. Two of the 250 mg tablets should be taken 4 times a day for 10 days.

Syphilis has an incubation period of 2 to 6 weeks before the characteristic sore appears. This appears as a painless ulcer (¼ to ½ inch), generally with enlarged, nontender lymph nodes in the region. Special lab tests on the patient's blood will be necessary to identify this disease and a special microscopic examination of a scraping of the lesion can be diagnostic. This lesion may not appear in a syphilis victim, making the early detection of this disease very difficult. A second stage consisting of a generalized skin rash (generally, which does not itch, does not produce blisters and frequently appears on the soles of the feet and hands) appears about 6 weeks after the lesions mentioned above. The third phase of the disease may develop in several years, during which nearly any organ system in the body may be affected. The overall study of syphilis is so complicated that a great medical instructor once said, "To know syphilis, is to know medicine."

The treatment of syphilis is also with penicillin, namely an injection of 1.2 million units of Benzathine Penicillin. However, an alternate therapy is also the use of the Sumycin, again two 250 mg tablets taken 4 times a day. This should be continued for 15 days. The patient should be checked by a physician when the expedition is completed to make sure that blood studies show syphilis was completely eradicated.

The best course of action when a patient apparently has contacted gonorrhea or suspects contact with syphilis is to treat with the drug available in your kit (i.e., Sumycin) for the full 15 days. This will help insure that a hidden case of syphilis has been ablated. If this type of fooling around is anticipated, make sure that the antibiotic quantity is sufficiently large to allow such liberal amounts to be dispensed. The best treatment is prevention, and the best prevention is abstention. Easy said.

ROCKY MOUNTAIN SPOTTED FEVER -- This is an acute and serious infection caused by a microorganism called *Rickettsia rickettsii* and transmitted by Ixodid (hardshelled) ticks. This same tick family also spreads Colorado Tick Fever. It is most common in the states of North Carolina, Virginia, Maryland, the Rocky Mountain States, and the state of Washington. There were 700 cases of this disease in 1976 with peak incidence from May to September.

Onset of infection is abrupt, after a 3 to 12-day incubation period (average 7 days from the tick bite). Fever reaches 103° to 104°F within two days. There is considerable headache, chills, and muscle pain at the onset. In four days a rash appears on wrists, ankles, soles, palms, and then spreads to the trunk. Initially pink, this rash turns to dark blotches and even areas of hemorrhage or bleeding under the skin that can form ulcers in severe cases.

Any suspected case of Rocky Mountain Spotted Fever should be considered a MEDICAL EMERGENCY. *Do not wait for the rash to develop,* rather start the patient on the antibiotic from the Rx medical kit. Give Sumycin 250 mg., two tablets every 6 hours and keep on this dosage schedule until the total time from the onset of the disease is 14 days. This is a drug of choice and its early use can cut the death rate from 20% to nearly zero. Do not wait for the rash to appear or a firm diagnosis to be made. The sooner the antibiotic is used, the greater the chance for total recovery. Prevention is by the careful removal of ticks, the use of insect repellant and protective clothing, and/or the use of a specific vaccine as described on pages 97 and 104.

COLORADO TICK FEVER -- A viral disease spread by Ixodid (hard-shelled) ticks, this disease is 20 times more common than Rocky Mountain Spotted Fever in Colorado. It is also found in the other states of the Western Rocky Mountains and provinces of Western Canada. It is most frequent in April-May at low altitudes and June-July at high altitudes.

Onset is abrupt, with chills, fever of 100.4° to 104°, muscle ache, headache, eye pain, and eye sensitivity to light (photophobia). The patient feels weak and nauseated, but vomiting is unusal. During the first two days, up to 12% of victims develop a rash. In half the cases the fever disappears after two to three days and the patient feels well for two days. Then a second bout of illness starts which lasts intensely for two to four days. This second phase subsides with the patient feeling weak for one to two addtional weeks.

This disease requires no treatment other than bed rest, fluids to prevent dehydration, and medications to treat fever and aches. However, as the same ticks can also spread potentially dangerous Rocky Mountain Spotted Fever, treatment with Sumycin as described in that section should be started immediately and this therapy continued for 14 days. This should be accomplished without waiting for the characteristic rash of Rocky Mountain Spotted Fever or the fever pattern of Colorado Tick Fever to develop or for a firm diagnosis of either to be established by a physician.

LACERATIONS -- In all lacerations the first order of business is stopping the bleeding. This is best done with pressure -- in fact, pressure alone will stop bleeding from amputated limbs! The first thing available is frequently the human hand. Press tightly against the wound. When better organized, remove your bloody hand and place a sterile gauze against the laceration. The best item in your kit is the Povidone-iodine Prep Pad to scrub out the wound. This, unfortunately, will restart the bleeding. After the scrubbing process, again stop the bleeding with direct pressure. Dry the skin on either side of the laceration and place butterfly bandages across the wound to pull skin edges together. Pinch the wound edges together while applying the butterfly strips to obtain the best approximation (see *Figure 11*).

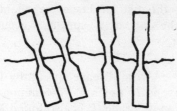

FIG. 11

BUTTERFLY BANDAGES

The commercial butterflies are superior to homemade in that they are packaged sterile with a no-stick center portion. They can be made in the field by cutting and folding the center edges in to cover the adhesive in the very center of short tape strips, thus avoiding tape contact with the wound. Of course, such homemade strips will not be sterile, but in general, will be very adequate.

The wound should be lightly coated with triple antibiotic ointment (a nonprescription item) and covered with a light gauze dressing. Change dressings whenever they become wet, as dampness will increase the likelihood of infection and also cause the butterfly strips to fall off. If these strips do become unattached, wipe the skin surface dry, taking care not to disturb the wound, and reapply.

Giving a prophylactic antibiotic by mouth is generally not required, and if none is available the patient can be expected to do very well with wound cleansing, irrigation and a light coating of the triple antibiotic ointment. When in the wilderness, however, I would provide systemic antibiotic coverage for the first 4 days with the Sumycin 250 mg, 1 tablet 4 times a day from the prescription kit. If weight permits, the inclusion of Hibiclens Surgical Scrub would be ideal. Manufactured by Stuart Pharmaceuticals, its onset of action is rapid and its duration of effectiveness is far longer than Povidone-iodine surgical scrub or Hexachlorophene surgical scrubs. It is currently available in the United States without a prescription.

If the laceration can possibly be held together (approximated) with tape, by all means use tape as the definitive treatment. Butterfly bandages are ideal. If taping will not hold the wound closed -- and this may be the case when a stretch is placed frequently on the wound due to its location -- then it will have to be sutured (stitched). Suture material is available in many forms and with many different types of needles.

For the expedition medical kit, I would recommend using 3-0 Ethilon Suture with a curved pre-attached FS-1 needle. This comes in a sterile packet ready for use. It will be necessary to use a needle holder to properly use this suture. The needle holder looks like a pair of scissors, but it has a flat surface with grooves that grab the needle and a lock device that holds the needle firmly. It is held as illustrated (see *Figure 12*) to steady the hand.

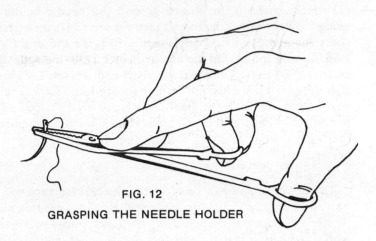

FIG. 12

GRASPING THE NEEDLE HOLDER

Apply pressure in the direction of the needle, namely twist your wrist in such a manner that the needle will press directly against the skin and cleanly penetrate, following through with the motion to allow the needle to curve through the subcutaneous tissue and sweep upward and through the skin on the other side of the wound. (Note illustration *Figure 13*).

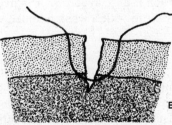

FIG. 13

PROPER PLACEMENT
OF SUTURE

EQUAL DEPTH ON BOTH SIDES OF CUT.

It is important to have the needle enter both sides of the wound at the same depth or the wound will not pull together evenly and there will be a pucker if the needle took a deep bite on one side and a shallow bite on the other (see *Figure 14*).

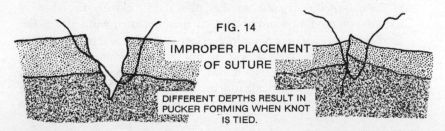

FIG. 14

IMPROPER PLACEMENT
OF SUTURE

DIFFERENT DEPTHS RESULT IN
PUCKER FORMING WHEN KNOT
IS TIED.

A square knot is tied with the use of the needle holder in a very easy manner. Loop the suture around the needle holder once, using the long end of the thread (see *Figure 15A*), then grasp the short end and pull the wound together (*Figure 15B and C*). Then loop the long end around the needle holder again the opposite way (*Figure 15D*) and again grasp the short end (*Figure 15E*) and pull tight (*Figure 15F*). This will form a square knot. Repeat this process a third time in the original direction to insure a firm knot. Do not pull too tightly as this will pucker the skin, just an approximation is required. Frankly, a knot tied in any fashion will do perfectly well.

The entrance and exit point of the needle puncture will bleed quite well usually. A little pressure will always cause this bleeding to stop -- it is not even necessary to delay your sewing to even worry about it -- just reclean the wound when you are done to remove dried blood, apply pressure until this bleeding from the needle punctures stops and dress the wound as indicated above. Suture through the skin surface only and avoid important structures underneath. If tendon or nerve damage has occurred, irrigate the wound thoroughly with the cleanest water available, scrub out as indicated above and repair the skin wound with either tape or stitches as necessary. The tendon, etc., can be repaired by a surgeon upon return to the outside -- weeks later *if necessary*. In fact, after a tendon laceration if a delayed repair is necessary, the surgeon would probably want to wait a week to make sure that no infection is going to develop.

For anesthesia you will probably want to use 2% Xylocaine. This will require a Rx for the medication and the syringe and needle to administer it. Inject through the wound, just along under the skin on both sides of the cut. This is probably not necessary, however, because the pain of the injection is hardly less than just sewing the wound up in the first place and the wilderness may justify the cruel appoach of no local infiltration, due to the problem of carrying the injectable medication and syringe.

These stitches should not be placed too closely together -- usually, on the limbs and body 4 stitches per inch will suffice. On the face, however, use 6 per inch. Here it is best to use 5-0 Ethilon (with FS-2 needle), as it will minimize scar formation from the needle and suture. I use a 6-0 suture on the face, but it is considerably more difficult to use than the 5-0. The use of these stitches can be augmented with tape strips or butterfly closures to

FORMING A SQUARE KNOT USING A NEEDLE HOLDER

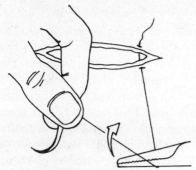

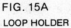

FIG. 15A
LOOP HOLDER

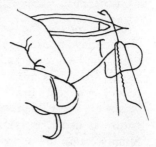

FIG. 15B
GRASP END THROUGH LOOP

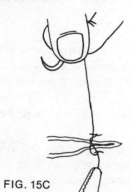

FIG. 15C
PULL TIGHT

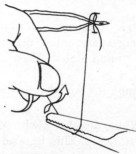

FIG. 15D
LOOP HOLDER IN REVERSE

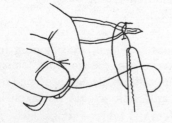

FIG. 15E
GRASP END THROUGH LOOP

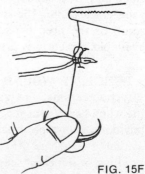

FIG. 15F
PULL TIGHT

help hold the wound together and to cut down on the number of stitches required. Once they are in, leave stitches in the limbs for 10 days, in the trunk and scalp for 7 days, and in the face for 4 days.

Lacerations on the tongue can almost always be left alone. The wound may appear ugly for a few days, but within a week or two there will be a remarkable healing. Infections in the tongue or the mouth from cuts are very rare; conversely, when a human bite occurs, it almost always gets infected. If a mouth laceration must be sewed, use a 3-0 plain gut suture (with FS-2 needle). This same suture is useful in tying off spurting blood vessels in wounds. Simply clamp the spurting vessel with the needle holder and tie the flesh pinched at the tip of the needle holder with the plain gut suture with a square knot or any knot that you can manage. Another person may have to hold the needle holder and remove it for you when doing this.

It is interesting to note that the purchase of needle holder, hemostat and suture material can be done without a prescription in the United States. These items can be bought from the publisher and a price list will be sent upon request. The Xylocaine and syringe for injection will have to be obtained with a prescription.

While in the bush you will want to cold sterilize your instruments. This is done by thoroughly wiping them with the Povidone-iodine prep pad. The adherent material can then be wiped off with an alcohol prep pad just prior to use. Have a very clean or sterile bandage to lay the instruments on when preparing your surgical site. The surgeon *must* clean his hands with surgical scrub or the prep pads. As mentioned, the best surgical scrub available currently is probably Hibiclens.

PUNCTURE WOUND -- Allow these to bleed, thus hoping to effect an automatic irrigation of bacteria from the wound. Cleanse the wound area with surgical scrub, or with an alcohol prep pad or povidone iodine prep pad. An oral antibiotic should be taken if available -- such as (Rx) Sumycin 250 mg, 1 tablet 4 times daily. If swelling or infection seem to have ensued, start warm soaks, thus hoping to draw infection to the surface. These soaks should be applied for 15 minutes, 4 times daily; make them as warm as the patient can tolerate without burning him. Larger pieces of cloth work best -- such items as undershirts -- which should be cleaned

with hot water and soap after each use. Apply triple antibiotic ointment and bandage between soaks. If this swelling continues to increase, treat as discussed under ABSCESS.

FISHHOOK -- The easiest method of removing an imbedded
fishhook, is to push the hook the rest of the way through the skin,
following the natural curve of the hook, then cut off the barb and
pull the hook back through the original wound (see *Figure 16*). A
pair of side cutting wire cutters should be included in every fishing
tackle kit, just for this purpose.

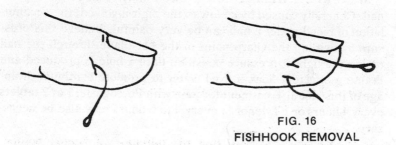

FIG. 16
FISHHOOK REMOVAL

If the Rx medical kit is along, a small injection of 2% Xylocaine
(about .2 ml) can be used to numb the skin at the point that the
barb is about to be shoved out. This will make the procedure pain
free. Treat this wound as described under PUNCTURE WOUND,
Page 80. As Calvin Rutstrum mentioned, if this hook removal process may endanger any vital structure, secure the hook's position
with tape and evacuate the patient to a physician.

SPLINTER -- Prepare the wound with povidone-iodine prep pad
or alcohol prep pad. The latter may be best as it does not discolor
the wound and disguise the splinter, if minute. If the splinter is
shallow and the point buried, using a needle or #11 scalpel blade,
tease the tissue over the splinter to remove this top layer. The
splinter can then be pried out better.

It is best to be aggressive in removing this top layer and obtaining a substantial bite on the splinter with the splinter forceps (or
tweezers), rather than nibbling off the end when making futile attempts to remove with inadequate exposure. In using the splinter
forceps, grasp the instrument between the thumb and forefinger,
resting the instrument on the middle finger and further resting the
entire hand against the victim's skin, if necessary, to prevent
tremor. Approach the splinter from the side, if exposed, grasping
as low as possible. Apply triple antibiotic ointment afterwards.

Tetanus immunization should be up to date. If the wound was apparently dirty, start the victim using hot soaks applied to the wound for 15 minutes, four times a day, to help draw possible infection, applying the antibiotic ointment (from either the Rx or nonRx kit) after each soak. If infection becomes apparent (swelling increases, redness and pus drainage), start the patient on two Sumycin, 250 mg tablets, four times a day, until symptoms abate. Continue the hot soaks during this time. See the section on PUNCTURE WOUNDS.

SUBUNGUAL HEMATOMA -- Blood under a fingernail or toenail. Generally caused by a blow to the digit involved, the accumulation of blood under a nail can be very painful. Relieve this pressure by twirling the sharp point of the #11 blade through the nail (using the lighest pressure possible) until a hole is produced and draining effected. Soak in cool water to promote continual drainage of this blood. Treatment for pain with Percogesic, 1 or 2 tablets every 4 hours or 1 Tylenol #3 every 4 to 6 hours may also be necessary.

INGROWN NAIL -- This painful infection along the edge of the nail can, at times, be relieved with warm soaks and antibiotic and pain medication as mentioned under the section PARONYCHIA (see *Figure 17*). However, it will probably have to be surgically corrected by infiltrating the involved side with 2% Xylocaine (2 ml generally suffices), including the nail bed.

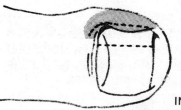

FIG. 17
INGROWN NAIL

This infiltration is a very painful procedure, but it does provide complete pain relief if enough is injected. Cut the nail about 1/3 of the way in from the involved edge using the operating scissors (ideally). This cut should be extended under the skin at the base of the nail. Grasp the sliver of nail, thus cut free from the remaining nail, using the needle holder with as deep a bite as possible. This action will cause separation of the grasped sliver from its attachment to the nail base. A considerable pull is required. If granulation tissue (proud flesh) has formed along the involved side, as it frequently has, this should ideally be cut away using the #10 scalpel. A simple wedge of this tissue is removed.

Dress between soaks with triple antibiotic ointment. Remove bandages when soaking.

PARONYCHIA -- or infection of the nail base. This very painful condition should initially be treated with warm soaks, 15 minutes 4 times a day and the use of oral antibiotics (such as Rx Sumycin 250 mg, 4 times daily) and pain medication. If the lesion does not respond with 2 days, or if it seems to be getting dramatically worse, an aggressive incision in the region of the swelling behind the nail with a #11 blade will be necessary (see *Figure 18*). This wound will bleed freely -- allow it to do so. Change bandages as necessary -- and continue the soaks and medications as described above.

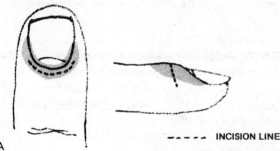

FIG. 18
PARONYCHIA

- - - - - INCISION LINE

ABSCESS or BOIL -- Apply heat 15 minutes 4 times a day to draw to a head. Do not squeeze, allow to drain spontaneously -- especially if it appears on the face. Other than on the face, once a head has formed, this should be lanced with a Bard Parker #11 scalpel (see *Figure 1*).

An abscess should be managed by a physician, if at all possible. Do not open until the head on the surface feels soft. Make the incision into the abscess deep enough to enter the pus filled cavity beneath the surface. A mixture of blood and pus will generally spew out, as the abscess is generally under pressure. They are also frequently loculated, consisting of several individual pockets within the walled-off abscess area. These locules will need to be opened -- probably the best way is to insert a hemostat, plunging it into the four quadrants of the wound, and opening the mouth to break down the walls of the internal locules. This is a very painful procedure. It should be completed in 15 seconds.

Do not squeeze on the boil, as this may force the material to dissect deeper and spread the infection. Continue hot soaks and change dressings as required. Remove dressings when applying the hot, wet soaks. The cloth used for the soaks will have to be thoroughly cleaned with hot water and soap between uses. It need not be sterile.

This incision and draining will frequently cure an abscess, even without oral antibiotics. From the Rx kit, give Sumycin 250 mg, 2 tablets every 6 hours for two to three days, then 1 tablet every 6 hours until the lesion has disappeared. Cover the wound between soaks with a coating of triple antibiotic ointment (nonRx) and sterile gauze.

FELON -- a deep infection of a finger tip is called a felon. Treatment is effected by a very aggressive incision, called a fish-mouth incision, made along the tip of the finger from one side to the other and extending deep to the bone! (See *Figure 19.*)

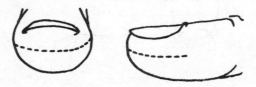

----- INCISION LINE

FIG. 19

FELON

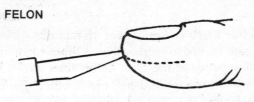

The pain is severe and not helped by injection of Xylocaine. But relief is quick in coming as pressure from the pus build-up is then alleviated. Allow this wound to bleed freely. Soak in warm water for 15 mintues, 4 times daily. Give oral pain medication -- nonRx Percogesic 2 tablets every 4 hours, or Rx Tylenol #3, 1 tablet every 4 hours. Also start the victim on antibiotic, Sumycin 250 mg tablets, 2 tablets every 6 hours for the first 2 to 5 days, then 1 tablet every 6 hours until the lesion is healed. Give the first dose of pain medication and antibiotic one hour before making the incision.

BLISTERS -- Blisters form in the skin surface from friction or thermal injury. If they are on a nonpressure area, they would best be left alone and protected from puncture, as the skin forms an excellent barrier against infection.

If it is painful, on a pressure bearing surface, or interferes with function or may burst due to size and location, it should be lanced. Clean the blister and the surrounding tissue with povidone iodine prep pad or alcohol prep pad and lance with a sterile #11 Bard Parker scalpel blade. Lance the blister at a bottom edge with a large enough incision so that the contents can be gently squeezed out with pressure using a sterile gauze pad. Once opened, this wound will have to be protected against infection with triple antibiotic ointment (nonRx) and sterile dressings. Do not remove the blistered skin for three to five days, thus allowing the skin beneath to mature. The deflated blister skin will still provide a protective coating for the delicate under-layer. Prevent friction blisters by covering hot spots with bandage plastic strips, tape or ideally moleskin. Protect the formed friction blister by cutting a donut out of moleskin, placing it around the afflicted area, and covering the top with a sterile dressing.

FUNGAL INFECTIONS -- They can be expected when there is itching, redness, and at times skin eruptions ranging from small blisters to dry scaly skin -- principally located between the toes (tinea pedis -- athlete's foot), in the groin (tinea cruris -- jock itch), or in circular patches on the body (tinea corporis -- body ring worm). Skin rashes can be a dilemma when it comes to their proper identification, even for an experienced physician. The best nonRx medication for fungal treatment is 1% tolnaftate (Tinactin Cream) -- it is virtually non-sensitizing and does not ordinarily sting or irritate intact or broken skin. This preparation would do no harm if applied to a nonfungal lesion (such as a contact dermatitis -- poison ivy), so when the body location appears suspicious, it would be perfectly all right to institute therapy until a physician can be consulted.

At times, home therapy can confuse the dermatologist because of inadvertant changes made in the lesions. This preparation will not disguise a lesion or confuse a dermatologist later. Just inform him that you have been using it. Most laymen are able to correctly identify athlete's foot and jock itch; many of them are aware of its chronic nature and the frequent flare-ups that are possible. If a member of your party is frequently bothered by one of these maladies, it would pay to add a 1/2 ounce tube of Tinactin to the expedition medical kit. Make sure that socks and clothes in contact with the lesion are not exchanged on the trip.

TENDONITIS -- The most common reason for development of tendon inflammation or tendon sheath inflammation is over-use of a particular muscle group and tendon. The ancient French trapper frequently encountered an Achilles tendonitis while snowshoeing, which they aptly termed "Mal de racquette". Persons hammering, axing, or playing tennis are familiar with epicondylitis of the elbow, which is inflammation of a bursa (or lubricating sack in the elbow). Cave explorers and canoeists will, on occasion, encounter a patellar bursitis in a knee, and many people have formed bursitis flare-ups in a shoulder due to repeated use of certain arm action.

The best medication in the medical kits for therapy of these problems is a good old-fashioned aspirin. 10 grains taken every 4 to 6 hours may be necessary. (The average tablet is 5 grain.) Generally the application of heat to the area helps calm down the irritation, but at times this makes the pain worse -- in which case cold compresses should be tried. Avoid making the movements which seem to cause the most pain for 5 to 7 days. If one is not careful, particularly with some shoulder flare-ups, continued lack of use may cause the shoulder to "freeze up" and loss of function can result.

Certainly range of motion may be started after 1 week without harm. Non-steroid anti-inflammatory agents stronger than aspirin may be indicated, particularly when the action must be continued on an expedition. A useful alternative drug is indomethacin 50 mg taken 4 times daily, or oxyphenbutazone 100 mg taken 4 times a day. For the most part, however, aspirin is very effective, costs less, and has less side effects. The main side effect of the two alternative drugs mentioned is severe heartburn -- these medications should be avoided in anyone with ulcer history. In fact, aspirin itself should be used only with care in these people -- generally on a full stomach only.

FRACTURES -- Broken bones are a source of much concern when in isolated areas. Each fracture has several critical aspects in its management to consider: 1) loss of circulation or nerve damage if bone spicules are pressing against these structures due to deformity of the fracture; 2) induction of infection if the skin is broken at or near the fracture site; 3) proper alignment of bone fragments so that adequate healing takes place.

At times it will be uncertain whether or not a fracture actually exists. There will be point tenderness, frequently swelling and discoloration over the fracture site or the generalized area, and in obvious cases, deformity and loss of stability. If doubt exists, splint and treat for pain, avoiding the use of the involved part. Within a few days the pain will have diminished and the crisis may be over. If not, the suspicion of fracture will loom even larger.

With proper splinting, the pain involved with a fracture will decrease dramatically. Pain medication should be provided as soon as possible. From the nonRx kit, 2 Percogesic every 4 hours may be necessary, especially in the early stages. The muscle relaxant properties of Percogesic will help relieve the terrible muscle spasm that accompanies many fractures and dislocations or, with the Rx kit, provide 2 Tylenol #3 every 4 hours; this may be boosted with 1 Phenergan, 25 mg every 4 hours to augment the effect of the pain medication and to provide some muscle relaxation.

Reduction of fractures should be left to the hands of skilled persons -- a minimum of common sense, however, can be applied to minimize the damage and to make temporary repairs until a physician can be consulted later. The adage "splint them as they lie" is the golden rule in handling wilderness fractures. However, if obvious circulation damage is occurring, namely the pulses distal to the fracture site have ceased, the extremity is turning blue and cold to touch, or numbness is apparent in a portion of the limb distal to the fracture, severe angulations of the fracture should be straightened to attempt to eliminate the pressure damage. Broken bone edges can be very sharp -- in fact a laceration of the blood vessels and nerves may have already occurred, thus causing the above symptoms. An attempt at correcting alignment may cause further damage, thus the recommendation to "splint them where they lie". Splints must be well padded to prevent skin damage. Pneumatic splints are available from any outfitters. Fracture splinting is generally well covered in first aid courses. Such a course should be taken prior to any major expedition into the bush. Improvisation is the name of the game in fracture immobilization and having an adequate first aid course provides one with information upon which to improvise. In general, fractures should be splinted in such a manner that the joint above and below the fracture site is immobilized.

HAND FRACTURES can generally be splinted with a cloth rolled in the hand, and the natural grip position of the hand assumed. This grip around the rolled cloth can then be wrapped with gauze to maintain the immobilization. **SHOULDER** injuries should be immobilized with a sling and another band tied around

88   WILDERNESS MEDICINE

the body to prevent movement. Fractures of the **THIGH** must be immobilized with a padded splint extending beyond the hip, with cloths wrapping the splint around the abdomen as well as the leg. An inner small splint is secured to the medial (inner) portion of the leg. (*See Figure 20*).

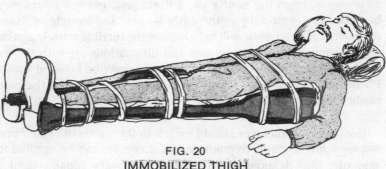

FIG. 20
IMMOBILIZED THIGH

Various traction devices can be improvised to overcome powerful muscle contractions of the thigh which will cause bone ends to override. A commercial device for this purpose is the Thomas splint, available through many medical/surgical suppliers. This device could not be justified except on major climbing expeditions or by rescue teams. Potential **NECK and BACK** injury is a particular reason for taking a first aid course. The management of these injuries can be fraught with disaster. The basic technique is immobilization. (*See Figure 21*).

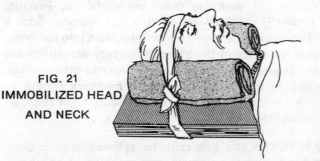

FIG. 21
IMMOBILIZED HEAD
AND NECK

A LACERATION or PUNCTURE WOUND AT THE FRACTURE SITE MEANS TROUBLE. Particularly if a spicule of bone is protruding. Wounds of this nature should never be sutured closed, as the incidence of severe infection is then greater. Cleanse the wound thoroughly, hopefully with the Hibiclens surgical scrub. Lacking that, with povidone iodine prep pads, alcohol prep pads, soap and water in decreasing order of effectiveness. Regardless of what is used, do a thorough job of cleansing. This will probably promote bleeding. The aggressiveness of this cleansing action should be done in such a manner as not to cause further damage, but certainly the area must be free of foreign particulate matter and as antiseptic as possible. Cover the wound with triple antibiotic ointment. Protect with sterile gauze dressings, with enough pressure to control bleeding only.

If the patient can be removed to a medical facility within two or three days, leave the bone specules protruding alone -- constantly keep the sterile dressing in place and moisten with boiled and cooled water. If no such evacuation is possible, after the very thorough cleansing as mentioned above, reduce the fracture with traction on both sides of the break to allow the best alignment possible. Dress wound as mentioned above. In all cases of laceration or puncture wound near the fracture, place the victim on oral antibiotics when available. From the Rx kit provide 2 Sumycin, 250 mg tablets every six hours until the return to civilization is completed. If no infection is apparent in ten days, the dosage may be decreased to one tablet every six hours.

FRACTURED RIBS -- may develop after a blow to the chest. A bad cough or sneeze may also crack ribs! There is point tenderness, exquisite pain with the lightest palpation over the fracture site. The pain at this site will be reproduced by squeezing the rib cage in such a manner as to put a stress across the fracture site. Deep breathing will also produce pain at that location. Treat with pain medication Rx Tylenol #3, one every four hours, avoid unnecessary movement, treat with antibiotic if a fever starts, Rx Sumycin 250 mg, two tablets every six hours.

It will not be necessary to strap or band the chest, except that such a band might prevent some rib movement and make the patient more comfortable. It is very important for the patient to breath and have some cough reflex to aid in pulmonary hygiene -- namely to prevent the accumulation of fluid in the lung which rapidly can lead to a pneumonia. Simply tying a large towel, an undershirt, etc. around the victim's chest should suffice. The fractured rib will take six to eight weeks to heal. A similar pain may be initially present due to a tear of the intercostal muscles or separation of cartilage from the bone of the rib, near the sternum or breast bone. These problems are treated as above. They heal much quicker, generally 3 to 5 weeks.

ANIMAL BITES -- Immediately wash with running water, canteen water or whatever else is available. Scrub the wound with povidone-iodine surgical scrub or disinfect the surface with povidone-iodine prep pads or alcohol prep pads. Animal bite victims should have had a tetanus toxoid immunization within the previous 5 years. If the skin surface has been punctured, it is best to start the victim on an antibiotic such as Sumycin 250 mg 4 times a day I would leave them on this for 4 days.

Punctures are best repaired only by taping with butterfly closures due to the high incidence of infection. Securing the closure with stitches may predispose an anaerobic infection starting. Regardless, if an infection does occur, take the tape strips off the wound and allow to drain. Soak the area in warm water -- or apply hot compresses for 15 minutes at a time, four times a day to promote draining and to draw the infection to the surface. If an abscess forms without drainage, open with the #11 stab blade scalpel to allow the pus to escape. (See section on ABSCESS.) Cover with sterile dressings which may be removed during the soaking process. This opening and drainage and hot soaking process is even more important than the antibiotics. I have seen many cured of their abscesses with the incision and drainage, even though subsequent antibiotic studies showed that the medication they were taking was totally ineffective for the particular bacterium which grew from their wound culture. Prior to antibiotic therapy, this I&D (incision and drainage) technique was the victim's only hope. Certainly, use the antibiotic right after the bite to preclude this miserable experience, but if it fails, perform an I&D and double the amount of antibiotic to two 250 mg Sumycin tablets, four times a day, or preferably start a different antibiotic if available.

RABIES -- can be transmitted, on the North American continent, by several small mammals -- namely skunks, foxes, coyotes, wildcats, squirrels, and several species of bats. The time to be concerned is when bitten due to a nonprovoked attack. Obviously, if removing an animal from a trap, taking food from a critter, or separating mother from child causes a fierce attack and bite, rabies would be of virtually no conern. Being bitten by a wounded animal is a little more questionable -- the animal may have fallen from a tree due to incoordination caused by rabies.

Under questionable conditions, treat the victim with a thorough cleansing as mentioned in the section on ANIMAL BITES. Start antibiotic to prevent bacterial infections; the patient had then better report to a physician for rabies immunization within two weeks. If more time elapses, the patient may have to be treated with not only the rabies vaccine, but also the rabies antiserum (which, unfornately is made from horse serum and is therefore rather tricky to use -- just as the snake antivenin). It will generally be impossible to preserve and return for analysis the carcass of the animal that did the biting -- it would similarly be rather difficult to capture and observe the animal for any period of time.

Rabies is a vicious disease that is generally fatal -- once symptoms start treatment is virtually hopeless. Because of this, there is generous use of the rabies vaccine. Persons having to work with potentially rabid animal populations can be immunized with the vaccine and given yearly booster shots. It is possible to obtain the disease by merely being contaminated with the saliva or blood of an infected animal -- possibly even by breathing in dust infected with the virus (such as in an infected cave).

BEE STINGS (also Wasp, Yellow Jackets, Hornets) (Hymenoptera) -- Stings from these insects hurt instantly and the pain lingers. The danger comes from the fact that many persons are "hypersensitive" to the venom and can have an immediate "anaphylactic" shock which is life-threatening.

The pain of the sting may be stopped with local application of cold, application of a paste of baking soda/water slurry, or a topical anesthetic such as dibucaine 1% ointment from the nonRx kit or Pontocaine .5% (ophthalmic) from the Rx kit. An aspirin, Percogesic, or (Rx kit) Tylenol #3 would also help with pain.

ANAPHYLACTIC SHOCK may occur within seconds in a very sensitive individual, or the shock may be preceded with welts and increasing respiratory distress. Anyone breaking out in welts after such a bite should be treated as if anaphylactic shock had occurred. The drug of choice is Adrenalin (epinephrine) 1:1,000 solution from the Rx kit (a component of the ANAKIT). The usual dose is .3 ml subQ (in the fatty layer beneath the skin). This may have to be repeated in 15 to 20 minutes. From the nonRx kit also give chlorpheniramine 4 mg and repeat in 6 hours. If a steroid, such as dexamethasone (Decadron) is available, give 4 mg IM. A handy kit to take along is the Anakit*, made by Hollister-Stier Laboratories, consisting of prefilled syringe of epinephrine which can deliver two .5 ml doses and two 4 mg chlorpheniramine tablets. This kit is available by Rx only through a pharmacy. Other aspects of shock treatment, as described on Page 21 should also be observed.

*(Hollister-Stier Laboratories, Spokane, Wa. 99207 approximate retail price is $8.00)

SNAKE BITE -- The first problem is to determine if the bite was by a poisonous snake and if envenomation took place. If the snake was not seen, you will have to go on symptoms alone -- if your powers of identification are feeble, again you must rely on symptoms. The first symptom noted by many is a peculiar tingling in the mouth, often associated with a rubbery or metallic taste. This symptom may develop in minutes and long before any swelling occurs at the bite site. Envenomation may produce instant burning pain. Weakness, sweating, nausea and fainting may occur either with poisonous snake bites or nonpoisonous bites, simply due to the trauma of being bitten.

Poisonous snakes will generally leave fang marks (but it may be difficult to identify two perfect fang marks which are supposed to be so characteristic of the pit vipers -- the coral snake will not have fang marks, but will chew the victim and induce venom into the macerated tissue). With envenomation, within one hour there will generally be swelling, pain, tingling and/or numbness at the bite site. As several hours pass, ecchymosis (bruising) and discoloration of the skin begins and becomes progressively worse. Vesicles may form, sometimes the blisters are filled with blood. The superficial blood vessels may form clots or become thrombosed. This, in turn, could lead to sloughing and necrosis in several days. Chills and fever may begin, followed by muscle tremor, decrease in blood pressure, headache, blurred vision and bulging eyes.

With regard to the visual identification of the most common poisonous snakes in North America -- the Pit Vipers (Family Crotalidae) (rattlesnakes, copperheads and water moccasins), take their names from the deep pit between the eye and nostril, which is a heat-receptor organ. Most of them have a triangular head and they have a cat-like verticle elliptical pupil. Coral snakes (Micruruns fulvius) (Family Elapidae), while not pit vipers, also have the verticle elliptical pupils. Some nonpoisonous snakes do also. Color variation in coral snakes makes the old saying that if the "yellow is separated from the black, it is nonpoisonous" (i.e. not a coral snake, but a king snake, etc.), a very treacherous method of identification.

FIRST AID FOR SNAKE BITE -- NONPOISONOUS SNAKE BITES: Get away from the snake. Cleanse area with surgical scrub or alcohol prep pads -- apply suction to promote evacuation of puncture debris -- but no cuts. No constricting band. Cover with triple antibiotic ointment. Start Rx Sumycin 250 mg 4 times a day (or the alternate EES 400, 4 times a day), for 4 days to prevent infection. It is supposed that the victim has had his tetanus toxoid immunization.

PIT VIPERS BITE (not everyone bitten by a pit viper will have envenomation -- fully 20% with rattlesnakes and 30% of cotton mouth water moccasin and copperheads will not): DO NOT APPLY COLD -- this is associated with increased damage and death. 1) Immobilize the injured part at heart level in a position of function. 2) Place constriction band 2 to 3 inches above the bite site -- loose enough so that the finger can be placed beneath. It is important to allow blood flow. Simply, this is a constriction, not a tourniquet. 3) Reassurance, warmth, quiet, and evacuation to an MD. 4) If evacuation would take more than 1½ hours, immediately use incision and suction because 22% to 50% of the venom can be removed with this method if it is performed within 3 minutes -- lesser quantities if performed within 30 minutes. Make 2 small, parallel incisions, each through a fang mark if the latter are identifiable, 1/4 to 1/2 inch long and 1/8 inch deep. Apply suction for 15 to 20 minutes; at most 1/2 hour. Use suction cups from the various snake bite kits that are commercially available -- this may be done by mouth if the first-aider does not have oral cuts, loose teeth or other oral lesions (for his own safety). 5) Antivenin: Wyeth produces a polyvalent Crotalidae antivenin, which comes in a freeze-dried form, complete with a bottle of diluent and syringe assembly. This may be stored for fairly long periods at room temperature.

Each kit has a small bottle of horse serum to skin test the potential recipient, as the antivenin is made from horse serum. Many people are highly sensitive to the horse serum and it is possible that this antivenin preparation may be more lethal than the snake bite was for these people. The test dose of the horse serum must be kept refrigerated. It would seem that members of an expedition heading into potential poisonous snake-infested areas could ideally be tested for sensitivity to the horse serum prior to departure. This would then allow the administration to be made without waiting 15 minutes for a skin test. It would also allow the non-refrigerated transport of the antivenin sets. However, this is a bad idea as even skin testing can cause sensitization to develop in the individual and may result in anaphylactic (or immediate) shock upon giving the supposedly safe antivenin. I mentioned this idea, simply to warn against "thinking it up." A physician can order a special test called a radio-allergen immune assay -- it is safe and would indicate lack of sensitivity to horse serum. The use of the antivenin, and the quantities given are described in the brochure that comes with each ampule.

Generally, the minimal amount for an adult would be 3 amps, for a child 5 amps. For a swollen hand 5 to 8 amps IV initially, with another 8 ready to go if the swelling progresses. Severe envenomation may require over 38 amps! This antivenin is only available by prescription and the current wholesale drug cost is $20-$35 (1979)! Approximately 7 to 10 days later, recipients of so much horse serum will develop a delayed reaction called "serum sickness." This will generally have to be treated with antihistamines (such as the chlorpheniramine) and steroids. Steroids should not be used routinely in poison snake bites. 6) Start antibiotic such as Rx Sumycin 250 mg 4 times a day. 7) It is supposed that all trip members have current tetanus toxoid immunizations up to date.

CORAL SNAKE BITE -- 1) Wash the bitten area promptly and simply. 2) The eastern Coral Snake is leisurely about actually envenomating his victim, so rapid withdrawal from the attack may have resulted in no envenomation. 3) The other procedures -- except for rapid evacuation of the patient to the hospital -- are probably useless in this type of bite. 4) Some authorities would suggest a light constriction band both above and below the wound site. 5) Application of suction *without incision* would do no harm, but also would probably do no good. 6) Since the Coral Snake is an elapid, like the cobra, signs and symptoms of envenomation take time to develop and deterioration then proceeds so rapidly that the antidote may be of no avail. Many experts feel the antidote should be given immediately after skin testing in all cases. Most authorities feel two units of the Wyeth Micruris fulvis antivenin should be given IV immediately. Some would use 10 amps of the antivenin. 7) Protect from wound infection with the Sumycin 250 mg 4 times a day. 8) If respiratory distress ensues, respiratory assistance may have to be performed. If the symptoms progress to this point in the boondocks, survival is improbable. While a respirator in the intensive care unit of a hospital may pull a victim through, doing this manually is asking the impossible.

Snakebite prevention is easier than treatment -- wear boots that cover the ankle and avoid placing your hands or reaching into areas where your view is obstructed in habitats of poisonous snakes. Avoid poisonous snakes when seen, rather than trying to kill them. These steps will prevent most snake bite incidents from occurring.

SPIDER BITES -- Generally spiders will make a solitary bite, rather than several. If the person awakens with multiple bites, he has collided with some other arthropod most likely.

BLACK WIDOW -- (Latrodectus mactans) Generally a glossy black with a red hourglass mark on the abdomen. Sometimes the hourglass mark is merely a red dot or the two parts of the hourglass do not connect. At times the coat is not shiny and it may contain white. The bite may be only a pin-prick, but generally a dull cramping pain begins within one quarter of an hour and this may spread gradually until it involves the entire body. The muscles may go into spasms and the abdomen becomes board-like. Extreme restlessness is typical. The pain can be excruciating. Nausea, vomiting, swelling of eyelids, weakness, anxiety (naturally), pain on breathing may all develop. A healthy adult can usually survive, with the pain abating within several hours and the remaining symptoms disappearing in several days.

An ice cube on the bite, if available, may reduce local pain. A specific antidote is available. (L. mactans antivenim from Wyeth Drug Company), which should be given after skin testing to persons under 16 and over 65. A specific help in relieving the muscle spasm is 10 ml doses of calcium gluconate IV. For severe envenomation 10cc of methocarbamol IV is helpful or 10 mg of diazepam IV. In the wilderness nonRx first aid kit, the Percogesic 2 every 4 hours, or in the Rx kit Tylenol #3, 2 tablets every 4 hours and Phenergan 25 mg 2 tablets every 4 hours may be helpful.

BROWN RECLUSE -- (Loxosceles reclusa and related species) A brown coat with a black violin marking on the cephalothorax or top part of the spider; the initial bite is mild and may be overlooked at the time. In an hour or two, a slight redness may appear; by several hours a small bleb appears at the bite site. At times the wound begins to appear as a bull's eye with several rings of red and blanched circles around the bite. The bleb ruptures, forming a crust, which then sloughs off; a large necrotic ulcer forms wnich gradually enlarges. Over the first 36 hours, vomiting, fever, skin rash and joint pain may develop -- and hemolysis of blood may be massive.

There is no antidote for the venom. Early diagnosis is important since many of the problems can be avoided if the bitten area is literally excised, or cut out. This should be done during the first 8 hours by a physician -- if diagnosis is certain. Dexamethasone 4 mg IM every six hours during the acute phase is a steroid regimen that may also be of benefit, but the use of steroids after 48 hours may be of little help. The ulcerating lesion should be treated with triple antibiotic ointment. The use of this ointment and Percogesic may be the only remedy available to the average wilderness traveler. Or the Rx Wilderness Kit could provide Tylenol #3 every 4 hours for pain; Phenergan 25 mg every 4 hours to help with the nausea, pain and inflammation, and Cortisporin ophthalmic ointment every 4 to 6 hours for topical treatment. Other spiders may be confused with the Loxosceles. These may also produce edema and some tissue breakdown, but nowhere near the extent of the damage done by the Brown Recluse.

CENTIPEDE, MILLIPEDE, CATERPILLAR REACTIONS -- Millipedes and caterpillars do not bite, but they discharge a secretion that is irritating to the skin. These lesions should be washed off with soap and water. An ice cube will usually control the pain. Percogesic, one or two tablets every 4 hours may also be necessary. From the Rx kit, a single application of Cortisporin (ophthalmic) -- perhaps repeated in 8 hours, should suffice. Centipede bites may be similarly treated with the possible addition of chlorpheniramine 4 mg every 6 hours from the nonRx kit.

MOSQUITO -- To prevent bites, use a DEET (n, n diethyl-m-toluamide) product of 12% or greater. Netting is useful in infested areas. Electronic sound devices that repel these critters have never worked up North for me, but friends have found them useful in cave entrances in the lower 48 states.

Considerable numbers of bites, or sensitivity to bites, may require an antihistamine such as chlorpheniramine 4 mg, every 6 hours from the nonRx kit. Aspirin 5 grains every 4 hours is also a great itch reliever -- as itch is a specialized type of pain and travels along the same nerve fibers as pain. Dibucaine 1% ointment will relieve the itch. Vitamin B1 (thiamine) taken 100 mg a day for a week prior to departure and daily thereafter may lessen mosquito bites. The original work by Dr. Ray Shannon used 1/3 this dosage amount. I would be very interested in hearing reader comments concerning use of Thiamine (B1) as an insect repellent. See the section on ENCEPHALITIS on Page 100.

BLACK FLIES -- Prevention of bites will require frequent application of a DEET compound of 30% or stronger. Netting and heavy clothes may be required. They can cause nasty sores, which are usually self-limited although at times slow healing. If infection is obvious, use Sumycin 250 mg 4 times a day. Apply (nonRx) dibu-caine 1% ointment and (Rx) Cortisporin ointment or (nonRx) triple antibiotic ointment for skin care. See section on TULAREMIA Page 100.

TICKS -- In tick country frequently, at least daily, checks should be made of each other and of the individual trip member to ensure that these freeloaders are not attached. Besides passing on disease and an uncomfortable bite, they may also induce a paralysis -- which fortunately disappears once the tick is removed. This paralysis can be very difficult to diagnose until the tick is found and removal results in recovery.

A vaccine is available to prevent Rocky Mountain Spotted Fever, for those traveling into the endemic areas, North Carolina, Virginia, Maryland and in the Rocky Mountain states and Washington state. Apply a DEET product when traveling into tick country, consisting of 30% strength or greater. To remove, apply alcohol which may cause them to back out. Otherwise, heating an instrument, such as a needle, and applying may make them back off. Or one may grasp the head carefully with splinter forceps and remove. Avoid crushing the body or leaving the head behind.

CHIGGERS -- A very uncomfortable parasite, the old prevention was the application of flowers of sulfur, available at some pharmacies or high school laboratories. I have used this on many occasions in very infested areas and found that it works quite well. Or, apply a DEET product of 30% or better. Once afflicted, apply a spot of seam sealant, finger nail polish or other material that will suffocate the tick and eliminate their existence.

NO-SEE-UMS, Biting Gnats -- The scourge of the North Country. As they fly through the finest mosquito netting with ease, it is of no help. Apply a DEET product of 30% or greater concentration. When they are attacking, I have frequently rubbed myself with a wool blanket to eliminate some of the discomfort. Cold water helps. One remedy which I understand works quite well, but which I have never had along to try, is an application of Absorbine Jr!

SCORPION STING -- Most North American scorpion stings are relatively harmless. **Centruroides sculpturantus** resides in Mexico, Arizona, New Mexico and the California side of the Colorado River -- this scorpion is potentially lethal. A specific antivenin is available in Mexico. Besides extreme pain, paralysis may occur.

Further complications are severe high blood pressure and respiratory distress. With the common wilderness medical kit, little can be done except treat for pain. Due to the many complications of this bite, the patient should be evacuated to a hospital if at all possible.

ANT, FIRE ANT -- The latter can produce an intensely painful bite which will blister and take 8 to 10 days to heal. The greatest danger is to the hypersensitive individual who may have an anaphylactic reaction. This should be treated as indicated under BEE STINGS, ANAPHYLACTIC SHOCK section. Otherwise pain medication and use of Cortisporin ointment from the Rx kit, 1% dibucaine from the nonRx kit, or a topical treatment should suffice.

STINGING NETTLE -- This severe irritation can be instantly eliminated by an application of DEET insect repellent 70% concentration or better. I found this neat trick out the hard way (accidentally) while camping in fields of the stuff along the Cape Fear River in North Carolina. I have never seen this technique in print, but it works instantly.

POISON OAK, POISON IVY, POISON SUMAC -- The formation of a line of small watery blisters generally means a contact dermatitis due to a poisonous plant. A blush of the blisters or vesicles may appear at times. Treatment is with pain-killer to relieve the itch -- either ASA or Percogesic from the nonRx kit and chlorpheniramine 4 mg every 6 hours from the nonRx kit. Additional topical relief can be obtained by applying the dibucaine 1% (nonRx kit) every 6 hours or Cortisporin (Rx kit) every 6 hours.

POISONING, INGESTION OF POISONOUS PLANTS -- In the past two years, the Pittsburgh Poison Control Center managed the vast majority of their poison plant ingestion victims by treatment consisting of emesis (vomiting) induced by syrup of ipecac. This technique provided totally adequate therapy. 1/2 ounce of syrup of ipecac is given orally and two 8 ounce glasses of water follow to enhance the emesis. This technique provided superior emptying compared to gastric lavage (stomach pumping) and can even cause the expulsion of particles in the upper portion of the small intestine. If no vomiting occurs, repeat the dose of 1/2 ounce of syrup of ipecac in 20 minutes. If all fails, induce mechanical vomiting by gagging the throat with a finger or spoon. This latter technique may well be the only method available while in the bush.

SEA URCHIN -- The spiny processes from these can cause subsequent problems that are worse than the initial injury. The spines should be removed thoroughly -- a very tedious process. Vinegar or acetic acid soaks several times a day may help dissolve the spines that are not found.

JELLYFISH -- Tentacles can cause mild prickling to burning, shooting, terrible pain. The worse danger is shock and drowning, or hypersensitivity and anaphylactic shock. Avoid the use of hot water in treating this injury. First pour ocean water over the injury. Try to remove the tentacles with gloved hands. Pour alcohol (or ideally formalin) over the wound, which will prevent the nematocysts from firing more poison. Both ammonia or vinegar would work, but not as well as alcohol. Powder the area with a dry powder such as flour or baking powder. Gently scrape off the mess with a knife, but avoid cutting the nematocysts with a sharp blade. Next apply from the Rx kit Cortisporin and Pontocaine ointments. From the nonRx kit, one would apply the dibucaine ointment.

CORAL STINGS -- These injuries are treated as indicated under JELLYFISH.

CORAL CUTS -- Clean the wound thoroughly -- trivial wounds can later flare into real disasters that may go on for years. Clean thoroughly with a coarse cloth or soft brush and surgical scrub or soapy water. Then apply alcohol and finally hydrogen peroxide. This will help bubble out fine particles and bacteria. Apply Cortisporin ointment from the Rx kit (or triple antibiotic from the nonRx kit) and give Sumycin 250 mg 4 times a day from the Rx kit.

STING RAY -- The damage is done by the barbed tail, which lacerates the skin, imbedding pieces of the tail material and venom into the wound. The wound bleeds heavily, pain increases over 90 minutes and takes 6 to 48 hours to abate.

Immediately rinse the wound with sea water and remove any particles of the tail sheath visible, as these particles continue to release the venom. Hot water is the treatment of choice -- applied as soon as possible and as hot as the patient can stand it. The heat will destroy the toxin rapidly and remove the pain the patient is experiencing. After hot water has been applied and all tail particles removed, the wound may be closed with butterfly bandages or sutures. Elevation of the wound is important. If particularly dirty, leave the wound open and place the patient on Sumycin 250 mg 4 times a day from the Rx kit. Treat for shock as necessary.

SCORPION FISH -- Same treatment as STING RAY.

CATFISH STINGS -- Apply hot water as indicated under STING RAY. The wound must be properly cleaned and irrigated, using surgical scrub such as povidone-iodine. Place the patient on Sumycin 250 mg 2 tablets 4 times a day for several days to decrease the chance of wound infection, which is common with this injury.

ENCEPHALITIS -- Encephalitis from Group A Arbovirus (Western Equine Encephalitis, Eastern Equine Encephalitis, Venezuelan Equine Encephalitis) in Alaska, U.S., and Canada, and Group B Arbovirus (St. Louis Encephalitis) in the U.S. can be prevented by liberal use of repellent and covering exposed areas with netting or clothing to prevent bites from infected mosquitos. Symptoms of these illnesses include high fever (104°F) and generally headache, stiff neck and vomiting and, at times, diarrhea. These diseases can be fatal and require evacuation to medical help. Cool the patient with external means (cool water, fanning), and the use of aspirin or Percogesic. The disease occurs in epidemics; be very careful of mosquito exposure when the disease becomes prevalent.

TULAREMIA (Rabbit Fever; Deer Fly Fever) -- This disease can be contracted through exposure to ticks, deer flies, or mosquitos. It is also possible to have cuts infected when working with the pelts, or eating improperly cooked infected rabbits. Similarly, muskrats, foxes, squirrels, mice and rats can spread the disease via direct contact with the carcasses. Stream water may become contaminated by these animals.

An ulcer appears when a wound is involved and lymph nodes become enlarged first in nearby areas and then throughout the body. Pneumonia normally develops. The disease lasts 4 weeks in untreated cases. Mortality in treated cases is almost zero, while in untreated cases it ranges from 6% to 30%.

Treatment of choice is streptomycin, but Sumycin (tetracycline) suggested for the Wilderness Prescription (Rx) Medical Kit works extremely well. The average adult would require an initial dose of seven tablets (Sumycin 250 mg), followed by 2 tablets every 6 hours. Continue therapy for 5 to 7 days after the fever has been broken.

APPENDIX

IMMUNIZATION SCHEDULES

Immunization schedules for domestic and foreign travel are listed below. Due to the rapidly changing international requirements, it would be advisable to request the current copy of the booklet titled, HEALTH INFORMATION FOR INTERNATIONAL TRAVEL, U.S. Public Health Service, Superintendent of Documents, U.S. Government Printing Office, Washington, D.C. 20402 ($2.50 includes postage). The 20 most commonly required immunizations are listed below. Some of these schedules do not provide total protection, but they will then frequently ameliorate the disease. Prevention is a lot safer and less traumatic than attempting to cure a patient once in the field.

Other excellent publications for travelers going out of the U.S. or Canada are: FOREIGN TRAVEL IMMUNIZATION GUIDE by Hans Neumann, M.D. (revised yearly), Medical Economics Book Division, P.O. Box 554, Oradell, N.J. 07649 ($3.95 plus $1.00 postage); and HEALTH PRECAUTIONS FOR FOREIGN TRAVEL, by D. Blitz, available from the author, P.O. Box 2382, Boston, MA 02107 ($2.25 includes postage).

CHOLERA

Immunization consists of .5 cc injection followed in 1 month with a second dose of 1.0 cc. Smaller doses for children 9 and under are given. A booster dose of .5 cc every 6 months is required. This immunization provides 60 to 80% protection -- if obvious exposure is made, prompt prophylaxis with oral tetracycline may prevent infection (such as Sumycin 250 mg 4 times a day, or Vibramycin 100 mg 1 capsule daily). Effective 6 days after receiving shot, immediately, if booster.

Immunization is advisable for travel in parts of Asia, the Middle East and Africa.

INFECTIOUS HEPATITIS (HB Ag Negative, Hepatitis A, Short Incubation Hepatitis)

A single dose of pooled gamma globulin .02 to .04 ml of 10% solution per kilogram of body weight IM protects against or modifies hepatitis, an infection in exposed individuals. Travelers to zones of known poor sanitation should receive larger doses .06 to .12 ml per kilograms, to give protection for 5 to 6 months. This

101

should not be taken 6 weeks before or 2 week after receiving immunization with live virus or it may interfere with their effectiveness.

The common live virus vaccines are: small pox, yellow fever, polio, measles (rubeola) and German measles (rubella).

Effective protection is provided immediately.

INFLUENZA

Vaccines are prepared that give 1 to 2 years of immunity for prevalent strains of influenza A or B. New strains are constantly arising that require formulation of new vaccines to compensate for this "antigenic drift." Dosage is .5 cc IM in the fall of the year. Not required for routine expedition work, unless heading into epidemic area.

MALARIA

A vaccine has not yet been developed that has been proven safe and effective although several prototypes have received some publicity recently from the wire services. Regions of the world where malaria may be acquired are Africa, parts of Mexico and Central America, Haiti, parts of South America, the Middle East, the Indian subcontinent and Southeast Asia.

The recommended drug for most travelers is chloroquine (Aralen by Winthrop Laboratories) 500 mg, one tablet every week, starting one week before departure, continuing during the trip, and for six weeks after returning. In areas where malaria has become resistant to chloroquine (Southeast Asia, the Indian subcontinent, New Guinea, the interior of some South American countries, and Panama), the recommended prophylaxis is a combination of pyrimethamine and sulfadoxine (Fansidar, by Hoffman-La Roche) which is available only outside of the U.S.

For a current list of specific areas of risk one should send for a copy of INFORMATION ON MALARIA RISK FOR INTERNATIONAL TRAVELERS, by Sendihl ($2.40 plus $.50 postage), to the United Nations Bookshop, GA-32B, United Nations, New York, NY 10017.

PLAGUE

Immunization consists of 3 shots of .5 ml, .5 ml and .2 ml (in that order) about 4 weeks apart and boosters of .2 ml every 3 months while in endemic areas. This provides only partial protection. Immunization is required to all travelers to Southeast Asia. All three initial shots are necessary before entering the endemic area.

PNEUMOCOCCUS

A vaccine has been developed for high risk patients with chronic diseases or respiratory problems. One .5 ml injection is good for 3 years, and should not be repeated before that time. Routine use is not required.

POLIOMYELITIS

Active long term immunization is conferred with 3 doses of the Trivalent Oral Polyvalent Vaccine (TOPV). Up to 18 years of age, the full schedule would consist of 2 doses of TOPV by mouth 8 weeks apart, and a third dose 6 months to 1 year later. Anyone having a partial series may continue with the next dose(s), regardless of how long before the first (or second) dose was given.

Areas of increased risk include Mexico, Central America and South America. "Prior to travel to these areas, anyone who has completed the primary TOPV series in the past should be given a single additional dose of TOPV. Unimmunized adults should be given the full four dose series of injectable inactivated polio vaccine (IPV)(3 doses given at 1 to 2 month intervals, followed by a 4th dose six to twelve months after the third dose), if time allows or a minimum of two doses of IPV given a month apart. If less than a month remains prior to departure, the administration of a single dose of TOPV may be justified due to the potential high risk of exposure to wild poliovirus and the more rapid protective effect of TOPV."*

*Technical Bulletin, Indiana State Board of Health, Polio Immunization of Teenagers and Adults, Jan. 1979.

MENINGOCOCCUS

The vaccine should be used only under special circumstances (military personnel in the U.S. and persons traveling to areas of the world where meningococcal infection is epidemic).

RABIES

A pre-exposure regimen of duck-embryo rabies vaccine is approved for use for persons routinely exposed to potentially rabid animals -- including skunks, fox, raccoon and bats. Two techniques are in vogue. Either two 1 ml doses 1 month apart with another 6 months later, or three 1 ml doses weekly with a fourth 1 ml dose 3 months later. Titers should be drawn 3 to 4 weeks after the last injection to establish antibody response. Persons with continuous exposure should have booster doses (1 ml) every 2 to 3 years. Post-exposure regimen for previously unimmunized persons is outlined on Pages 90 and 91.

ROCKY MOUNTAIN SPOTTED FEVER
TICK FEVER; TICK TYPHUS - England
FIEBRE MANCHODA - Mexico
FIEBRE PETEQUIAL - Colombia
FIEBRE MACULOSA - Brazil

This disease is spread by ticks with most cases in the U.S. coming from the states of North Carolina, Virginia, Maryland, the Rocky Mountain states and the State of Washington. Immunization is available and valuable, but ease of treatment with antibiotics (tetracyclines, chloramphenicol) has decreased its use. In the areas of high tick exposure -- besides insect repellent and frequent tick removal checks -- the use of this vaccine is justified.

SMALLPOX

Vaccination is not required to enter the United States -- but is still a possible danger in a few countries such as Nepal, India, Pakistan, Bangladesh, Ethiopia and the Sudan.

Vaccination is required for entering several other countries. Again, check the current requirements in advance of travel. Vaccination provides immunity for 3 years, but travelers to those areas reporting outbreaks should obtain their vaccination within 6 months of departure.

It is possible that this disease may be truly irradicated from the face of the world -- but it has risen its ugly head several times since being declared extinct by World Health Organization officials several years ago.

Vaccination is effective 8 days after immunization; immediately in the case of a revaccination.

TETANUS -- DIPHTHERIA

All persons should have a tetanus booster every 10 years -- within 5 years for severe wounds or bites. Because of this, all trip personnel (regardless of destination), should have a booster current within 5 years. This can be given as tetanus-diphtheria toxoid, adult type -- to everyone 6 years of age and older.

Initial immunization consists of 2 doses of .5 ml 1 to 2 months apart and a third dose of .5 ml 1 year later.

TYPHOID

Immunization should be completed before heading into areas where typhoid is known to be epidemic, generally parts of Southeast Asia and Mexico. The vaccine is about 70% effective in preventing the disease and also decreases the severity of the disease.

Immunization consists of two .5 ml doses given subsequently 1 month apart. Effective for approximately 3 years, this should be boosted yearly in areas of high risk.

TYPHUS

A disease spread worldwide, it is prevented by eliminating lice and/or immunization with a specific vaccine. The disease is actually spread by lice feces. The vaccine may not provide full protection, but the disease in immunized people is much milder and of shorter duration. This disease is frequent after disasters; approximately three million people died of it during World War II.

Initial series is 2 injections 4 or more weeks apart. It is effective for 6 to 12 months and an injection booster is required at that time.

YELLOW FEVER

Immunization is required for travel to most countries in South America, Africa and Asia. The immunization consists of one .5 cc injection which confers immunity for 10 years. It is available only at designated Yellow Fever Vaccination Centers (check your local health department for the nearest facility).

Notes

Bibliography

American College of Surgeons, *Early Care of the Injured Patient*, 433 pages, W.B. Saunders, Philadelphia, **1976**.

American Heart Association, *CPR in Basic Life Support*, Dallas, **1974**.

American Pharmaceutical Association, *Handbook of Nonprescription Drugs, 5th Ed.*, 388 pages, Washington, D.C., **1977**.

Arena, J.M., MD, *Poisonous Plants*, Journal Continuing Education in Family Medicine, pages 13-25, July **1978**.

Babb, R.R., MD, *Travelers' Diarrhea*, Rational Drug Therapy, 10:1, Jan. **1976**.

Banyan Emergency Reference Guide, 8 pages, Banyan International Corporation, Box 1779, Abilene, TX 79604, **1978**.

Beeson, P.B., MD., et al, *Cecil Textbook of Medicine, 15th Ed.*, 2354 pages, W.B. Saunders, Philadelphia, **1979**.

Blitz, D., *Health Precautions for Foreign Travel*, P.O. Box 2382, Boston, MA 02107 ($2.25), 31 pages, **1978**.

Bonner, J.R., MD, *Stinging Insect Allergy*, Consultant, pages 49-55, Sept. **1978**.

Conn Current Therapy, Section 16, "Physical and Chemical Injuries", pages 869-884, W.B. Saunders, Philadelphia, **1978**.

Darvill, F., MD, *Mountaineering Medicine*, 52 pages, Skagit Mountain Resuce Unit, **1977**.

Emergency Medicine, *Immunization Update*, pages 24-33, Nov. **1978**.

Emergency Medicine, *Jaws that Bite, Things that Sting*, pages 25-59, July **1978**.

Etzwiler, D.D., MD, *When the Diabetic Wants to be an Athlete,* The Physician and Sportsmedicine, pages 45-50, Feb. **1974.**

Flint and Cain, *Emergency Treatment and Management,* 794 pages, W.B. Saunders, Philadelphia, **1975.**

Forgey, W.W., MD, *The Complete Guide to Trail Food Use, 2nd Ed.,* 112 pages, Indiana Camp Supply, Box 344, Pittsboro, IN 46167, **1977.**

Gray, W.D., *Poisonous Mushrooms and Mushroom Poisoning,* Drug Therapy, pages 103-112, Sept. **1978.**

Grey Owl, *Tales of an Empty Cabin,* 335 pages, Macmillan of Canada, Toronto, **1936.**

Glass, T.G., Jr., MD, *Early Debridement in Pit Viper Bites,* Journal of the American Medical Association, 235:2513-2516, June **1976.**

Gorde, W.N., MD, *Lightning,* Appalachian Trailway News, pages 17-19, Sept. **1978.**

Harkness, R., *OTC Handbook,* 134 pages, Medical Economics Company, Oradell, New Jersey, **1978.**

Houston, C.S., MD, *High Altitude Illness,* Journal of the American Medical Association, 236:2193-2195, Nov. **1976.**

Indiana State Board of Health, *Polio Immunization of Teenagers and Adults,* Technical Bulletin, Jan. 5, **1979.**

Kahn, F.H., MD, and Visscher, Barbara R., MD, *Water Treatment,* The Western Journal of Medicine, 122: 450-453, **1975.**

Kleiner, J.P., MD and Nelson, W.P., MD, *High Altitude Pulmonary Edema,* Journal of the American Medical Association, 234:491-495, Nov. **1975.**

Kodet, R., MD and Angier, B., *Being Your Own Wilderness Doctor,* 127 pages, Stackpole Books, Harrisburg, Pennsylvania, **1968.**

Lathrop, T., MD, *Hypothermia,* 29 pages, Mazmas, **1975.**

The Medical Letter, *Treatment of Frostbite,* Vol. 18, Dec. **1976.**

The Medical Letter, *Treatment of Snakebite in the U.S.A.*, Vol. 20, Nov. **1978.**

Medical News, *Chemical Sympathectomy May Aid Frostbite Patients*, Vol. 231, Jan. **1975.**

Medical Tribune, *Infection Control*, page 19, March **1977.**

Medical World News, *Protective Drugs Urged for Travelers to Malarial Areas*, pages 30-31, Jan. **1979.**

The Merck Manual, 13th Ed., 2164 pages, Merck and Company, Rahway, NJ, **1977.**

Moriarty, R.W., MD, *Poisonous Plants*, Drug Therapy, pages 101-109, July **1978.**

Nading, L., *Survival Cards*, Box 1805, Bloomington, IN 47402 ($2.50), **1976**

Nealon, T.F., Jr., MD, *Fundamental Skills in Surgery*, 327 pages, W.B. Saunders, Philadelphia, **1971.**

Neumann, H., MD, *Foreign Travel Immunization Guide*, 54 pages, Medical Economics Company, Oradell, NJ, **1979.**

Patient Care, *Update on Upper Airway Management*, pages 233-250, Sept. **1978.**

Petzoldt, Paul, *The Wilderness Handbook*, 286 pages, W.W. Norton and Company, New York, **1974.**

Physician's Desk Reference, 33rd Ed., 2047 pages, Medical Economics Company, Oradell, New Jersey, **1979.**

Rethmel, R.C., *Backpacking 6th Edition*, 232 pages, Follett Publishing Company, Chicago, **1979**

Reuler, J.B., MD, *Hypothermia: Pathophysiology, Clinical Settings and Management*, Annals of Internal Medicine, 89:519-527, Oct. **1978.**

Rowland, S., MD, *First Aid in Snakebite*, Consultant, pages 32-35, May **1978.**

Rutstrum, Calvin, *Chips from a Wilderness Log*, 234 pages, Stein and Day, New York, **1978**.

Rutstrum, Calvin, *New Way of The Wilderness*, 276 pages, Collier, New York, **1958**.

Rutstrum, Calvin, *Paradise Below Zero*, 244 pages, Collier, New York, **1968**.

Surgical Rounds, *Choke Prevention Methods Disputed*, page 47, Aug. **1978**.

Ward, Michael, MD, *Mountain Medicine*, 376 pages, Van Nostrand Reinhold Company, New York, **1976**.

Washburn, Bradford, *Frostbite*, 25 pages, Boston Museum of Science, **1974**.

Watt, C.H., MD, *Poisonous Snakebite Treatment in the United States*, Journal of the American Medical Association, 240:654-656, Aug. **1978**.

Wilkerson, J., MD, *Medicine for Mountaineering*, 2nd Ed., 368 pages, The Mountaineers, Seattle, **1975**.

Wolf, Harold, DrPH, Personal communication, Civil Engineering Dept., Texas A & M University, College Station, TX, **1979**.

THE PRESCRIPTION (Rx) MEDICAL KIT
For Extended Trips Where Medical Help Is Not Available

Ear ache   External infection (Hurts when pushing on tragus [nob at front of the outer ear)]

             Cortisporin (ophthalmic) ointment - apply 4 times daily - to melt with ear elevated and run in

             (If very severe with entire ear canal swollen shut):

             Sumycin tablets 250 - 1 tablet 4 times a day
             Tylenol #3 - 1 tablet every 4 hours for pain

      Middle ear infection (runny nose and head congestion present)

             Sumycin tablets 250 mg - 1 tablet 4 times a day
             Actifed - 1 tablet 4 times a day

Eye inflamed   Check for foreign body (speck). If foreign body seen, use:

             Pontocaine ophthalmic ointment .5% to deaden pain, remove foreign body with needle

      No foreign body, whites of both eyes inflamed - probably conjunctivitis

             Cortisporin ophthalmic ointment - small dab 4 times daily

Nasal congestion   Actifed - 1 tablet 4 times daily

Sore throat/laryngitis   Sumycin tablets 250 mg - 1 tablet 4 times daily for 10 days

Severe cough   Tylenol #3 - 1 tablet every 4 to 6 hours for cough

      With high temp add   Sumycin 250 mg - 1 or 2 tablets 4 times a day

Abdomen   Vomiting   Phenergan tablets 25 mg - 1 tablet every 6 hours

           Cramps &   Tylenol #3 - 1 tablet every 4 hours as needed
           diarrhea

           Heart   Camalox - 2 to 4 tablets, dissolved in mouth
           Burn

           Appendi-   Without medical help - move as little as possible
           citis   Tylenol #3 - 1 or 2 tablets every 4 hours for pain
                      Phenergan 25 mg - 1 tablet every 4 hours for nausea and to potentiate the Tylenol #3
                      Sumycin tablets 250 mg - 2 tablets every 4 hours
                      No food; small amounts of Gatorade, etc., as tolerated
                      Arrange for medivac by helicopter if possible; above steps only if no evacuation or outside help feasible

Constipation   Bisacodyl tablets 5 mg - 1 or 2 tablets; avoid with fruits in diet

Shock		Elevate feet, cover to keep warm; reassure; treat cause
	From bee sting	.3 cc epinephrine (Adrenalin) 1:1000 sub-Q from Anakit - also take chlorpheniramine from kit
Skin infection, dirty wound		Sumycin tablets 250 mg - 2 tablets 4 times dialy, decrease to 1 tablet 4 times a day after 4 days
		Open wound to drain pus; apply hot soaks 15 minutes 4 times daily
Cuts, burns		Cortisporin ophthalmic ointment - apply 3 to 4 times daily
	If severe	Add Sumycin tablets 250 mg - 1 tablet 4 times daily
Inflammation from insects		Phenergan tablets 25 mg - 1 tablet 4 times daily
	Or poison plants, itch	Cortisporin ophthalmic ointment - apply 3 to 4 times daily
	From fungus infection	Tinactin 1% - apply twice daily
Pain from tooth ache		Tylenol #3 - 1 or 2 tablets every 4 hours
	If severe	Add Phenergan tablets 25 mg - 1 tablet 4 times daily
Bladder infection or Urethral discharge		Sumycin tablets 250 mg - 1 tablet 4 times daily for 10 days Sumycin tablets 250 mg - 2 tablets 4 times daily for 10 days
Snake Bite	Non-Poisonous	Treat for shock; scrub wound with povidone-iodine prep pad; apply triple antibiotic ointment
	Poisonous	Treat for shock; apply constriction band; scrub lightly with povidone-iodine prep pad; apply suction immediately and continue for 30 minutes; if no evacuation possible, make parallel cuts 1/4'' by 1/2'' prior to suction. Dress wound with triple antibiotic; elevate limb - no ice!

DRUG AND SPECIAL EQUIPMENT LIST

Cortisporin ophthalmic ointment - 1/8th oz. tube
Sumycin tablets 250 mg - 80 tablets
Tylenol #3 tablets - 30 tablets
Actifed Tablets - 40 tablets
Pontocaine ophthalmic .5% - 1/8th oz. tube
Phenergan tablets 25 mg - 30 tablets
Xylocaine for injection 2% - 30 ml bottle 1 ea.
Syringe - 3.5 ml size, with 25 gauge needle, 2 ea.
Needle holder
Splinter forceps
Bandage scissors or operating scissors
Bisacodyl tablets 5 mg - 10 tablets
Aspirin, 5 grain - 25 tablets

Tinactin 1% 15 gram - 1 tube
3 packs of 5-0 ethilon suture (fine)
3 packs of 3-0 ethilon suture (heavy)
1 pack of 3-0 plain gut suture
10 povidone-iodine prep pads
1 Anakit
10 bandages 1'' x 3''; tape 1'' x 10 yds.
3 gauze pads 3'' x 3''
1 gauze roll 3'' x 10 yards
1 elastic bandage, 4'' x 5½ yards
10 Butterfly closures, medium
1 Moleskin 12'' x 2''
1 Cutter Snake Bite Kit

Sumycin is a tetracycline; it should not be given to children younger than 8 years and to women in the last half of pregnancy or who are nursing, or if allergy to this class of drug exists - a substitute would be Erythrocin ethyl succinate (EES 400), taken in the same dosage regimen as indicated above for Sumycin.

THE NONPRESCRIPTION (nonRx) MEDICAL KIT
For Extended Trips Where Medical Help Is Not Available*

Ear ache   External infection (Hurts when pushing on tragus [nob at front of the outer ear])

Schein Otic Drops - 4 drops every 4 hours
Triple antibiotic ointment - apply with Q-tip 3 times daily
Percogesic - 2 tablets every 4 hours for pain as needed
A prescription oral antibiotic should be taken

Middle ear infection (runny nose and head congestion present)

Chlorpheniramine 4 mg - 1 tablet 4 times daily
Pseudoephedrine 30 mg - 2 tablets 4 times daily
A prescription oral antibiotic should be taken

Eye inflamed   Check for foreign body (speck). If foreign body seen, use:

Percogesic - 2 tablets 1 hour before attempting removal
Yellow oxide of mercury 1% - apply every 4 hours

No foreign body, whites of both eyes inflamed - probably conjunctivitis

Yellow oxide of mercury 1% - apply every 4 hours

Nasal congestion   Chlorpheniramine 4 mg - 1 tablet 4 times daily
   & Sinus ache   Pseudoephedrine 30 mg - 2 tablets 4 times daily

Sore throat/laryngitis   Percogesic - 1 or 2 tablets every 4 hours for pain, fever

Severe cough   Hydrate; Percogesic, as above
With high temp, an oral prescription antibiotic should also be taken

Abdomen   Vomiting   Meclizine 25 mg - 1 tablet every 8 hours as needed

Heart   Camalox - 2 to 4 tablets, dissolved in mouth
Burn

Cramps   Bacid Capsules - 2 capsules every 4 hours as needed
and Diarrhea

Appendi-   Without medical help - move as little as possible
citis   Percogesic - 2 tablets every 4 hours for pain
Meclizine 25 mg - 1 tablet every 8 hours for nausea
No food; small amounts of Gatorade, etc., as tolerated
Prescription antibiotic coverage should be provided
Arrange for medivac by helicopter, if possible; above steps only if no evacuation or outside help feasible.

Constipation   Bisacodyl tablets 5 mg - 1 or 2 tablets; avoid with fruits daily in diet

Shock from bee sting		Elevate feet, cover to keep warm, constriction band above the sting site - before shock starts provide: Chlorpheniramine 4 mg - 2 tablets every 6 hours
Cuts, burns		Scrub wound with povidone-iodine prep pad Cover wound and 2°/3° burns with triple antibiotic oint.
Skin infection, dirty wound		Local heat, 15 minutes every 4 hours to raise abscess to a head; lance to allow draining - do not squeeze, continue hot soaks and dressing changes as required Pack abscess with povidone-iodine prep pad Triple antibiotic ointment on bandage with each change A prescription oral antibiotic should be taken
Inflammation from insects or poison ivy, itch		Chlorpheniramine 4 mg - 1 tablet 4 times daily Dibucaine ointment 1% - apply 2 to 3 times daily
From fungal infections		Tinactin Cream - apply 3 times daily
Pain		Percogesic - 1 or 2 tablets every 4 to 6 hours
Bladder infection		Push fluids - 8 quarts daily Acidify urine - cranberry juice, vitamin C, etc.
Snake Bite	Non-Poisonous	Treat for shock; scrub wound with povidone-iodine prep pad; apply triple antibiotic ointment
	Poisonous	Treat for shock; apply constriction band; scrub lightly with povidone-iodine prep pad; apply suction immediately and continue for 30 minutes; if no evacuation possible, make parallel cuts 1/4'' by 1/2'' prior to suction. Dress wound with triple antibiotic: elevate limb - no ice!

NONPRESCRIPTION DRUG AND SPECIAL EQUIPMENT LIST

Schein Otic Drops - 1 oz.	Triple antibiotic ointment - 15 packets
Yellow oxide of mercury ophth 1% - 1/8 oz.	Bacid Capsules - 20-30 capsules
Percogesic - 48 tablets	3 packs of 5-0 ethilon suture (fine)
Pseudoephedrine 30 mg - 50 tablets	3 packs of 3-0 ethilon suture (heavy)
Chlorpheniramine 4 mg - 25 tablets	1 pack of 3-0 plain gut suture
Needle holder	10 povidone-iodine prep pads
Splinter forceps	10 bandages 1'' x 3''; tape 1'' x 10 yds.
Wire Cutters, side cutting type	3 gauze pads 3'' x 3''
Bandage scissors or operating scissors	1 gauze roll 3'' x 10 yards
Bisacodyl 5 mg - 10 tablets	1 elastic bandage, 4'' x 5½ yards
Tinactin cream 1% - 1/2 oz.	10 Butterfly closures, medium
Camalox Tablets - 20 to 40 each	1 Moleskin 12'' x 2''
Dibucaine ointment 1% - 15 grams	1 Cutter snake bite kit
Aspirin, 5 grain - 25 tablets	20 Camalox tablets

*The items listed in this kit are available without prescriptions. The dosages and uses listed above, however, do not necessarily conform to the guidelines listed by the manufacturer, the FDA, or other agencies. The above use should be restricted to healthy young adults, not suffering from hypertension, diabetes, glaucoma, kidney disease, liver disease, thyroid disease, or ladies who are pregnant or nursing. Prior to embarking upon a wilderness expedition where such use of these items may be required, all participants should have a physical exam to insure their exclusion from the above categories.

CENTIGRADE-FAHRENHEIT CONVERSIONS

CENTIGRADE°		FAHRENHEIT°
FREEZING (WATER AT SEA LEVEL)		
0		32
26.5	CLINICAL RANGE:	79.7
27.0		80.6
27.5	DEATH	81.5
28.0		82.4
28.5		83.3
29.0		84.2
29.5		85.1
30.0		86.0
30.5		86.9
31.0		87.8
31.5	SEE PAGES 52-57	88.7
32.0		89.6
32.5		90.5
33.0		91.4
33.5		92.3
34.0		93.2
34.5		94.1
35.0		95.0
35.5		95.9
36.0	NORMAL	96.8
36.5		97.7
37.0		98.6
37.5		99.5
38.0		100.4
38.5		101.3
39.0		102.2
39.5	SEE PAGE 21	103.1
40.0		104.0
40.5		104.9
41.0		105.8
41.5		106.7
42.0	SEE PAGES 57-59	107.6
42.5		108.5
43.0		109.4
43.5		110.3
44.0		111.2
44.5		112.1
45.0		113.0
45.5		113.9
46.0	DEATH	114.8
46.5		115.7
47.0		116.6
BOILING (WATER AT SEA LEVEL)		
100		212

Instant Reference Clinical Index

Symptoms, regional anatomical or organ system involvement, therapy, diseases and traumatic conditions by common and scientific name, and medications by brand and generic name are listed and cross-referenced.

Page number in **bold** refer to principle listings.